EXPE
GUT BU

"Just look what you can do in fifteen minutes a day. This routine will get your stomach hard, tight and 'ripped.'"
   —**Bob Kennedy,** editor, *Musclemag International*

"Gut Busters is the best abdominal workout on the market. I use the exact plan described in it myself!"
   —**Gus Stefanidis,** Mr. Greece

"As a judge of bodybuilding contests, a bodybuilder, and a doctor of chiropractic, I must say *Gut Busters* will net an average man a champion's stomach in record time."
   —**Dr. Jack Barnathan,** Doctor of Chiropractic,
      Director of Sports Health Chiropractic, Bethpage, New York

"Joyce Vedral's workouts are always effective, and this one is no exception. Just take a look at the 'before and after' photographs, and you'll see what I mean."
   —**Andy Sivert,** Mr. North America, Mr. International

"The best workout and diet plan I've seen yet for strengthening the stomach, removing the excess fat, and producing hard, lean muscles. I will recommend this book to all of my patients."
   —**Jude Barbera, M.D.,** Assistant Professor of Surgery,
      Downstate Medical Center, Brooklyn, New York

"Gut Busters will give you a rock hard stomach in a matter of months."
   —**Lud Shusterich,** World Powerlifting record holder,
      member of the All Time Greats Bodybuilding Hall of Fame

more ...

"As a cosmetic surgeon, I strongly endorse this technique of working out as a way of looking well and maintaining the extremely important abdominal muscles which support the spine and back."

—**Dr. Gerald Acker, M.D., P.C.,** Director of Cosmetic Surgery, Long Beach Memorial Hospital, Long Beach, New York

"I will be eternally grateful to Joyce Vedral for putting my husband on the Gut Buster program. Just look what it did for him in three months' time! And not only that, by following the low-fat eating plan, he's been able to lower his cholesterol and his blood pressure as well."

—**Arlen Dash,** wife of Dave Dash,
see p. 22, "Before and After"

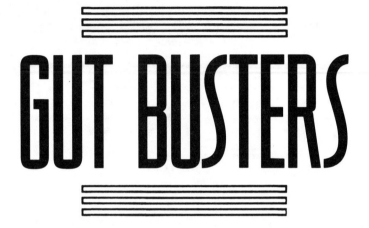

GUT BUSTERS

THE 15-MINUTE-A-DAY, 12-WEEK PLAN BY
JOYCE L. VEDRAL, PH.D.

FEATURING KENT MAURER

WARNER BOOKS

A Time Warner Company

*This book is dedicated to all of the wonderful men
who don't want to look like bodybuilders;
they just want to "get rid of their gut."*

*And to my "Uncle Dave," a "before" and "after" in this
book, for sticking with the program and proving that it
can be done at any age, despite a hectic schedule!*

———————————————————

The ideas, procedures, and suggestions contained in this book are not
intended as substitutes for consulting with your physician. All matters
regarding your health require medical supervision.

Kent Maurer appears on the cover of this book and in the inside
exercise photographs. He is currently Director of Cal-A-Vie Health Spa
in Vista, California.

Warner Books, Inc., 1271 Avenue of the Americas, New York, NY 10020

Ⓦ A Time Warner Company

Printed in the United States of America
First printing: February 1992
10 9 8 7

Library of Congress Cataloging-in-Publication Data

Vedral, Joyce L.
   Gut busters : the 15-minute-a-day, 12-week plan / by Joyce L.
Vedral ; featuring Kent Maurer.
      p.   cm.
   Includes bibliographical references.
   ISBN 0-446-39367-3
   1. Reducing exercises. 2. Abdomen—Muscles. I. Maurer, Kent.
II. Title.
   RA781.6.V43   1992
613.7′1—dc20   91-37871
                                                              CIP

Cover design by Julia Kushnirsky
Cover, back cover, and inside photography by Don Banks
Hair and makeup by Jodi Pollutro of Mike and Me Salon
Footwear for Kent Maurer by NIKE
Footwear for Joyce L. Vedral by Reebok
Book design by Giorgetta Bell McRee

Acknowledgments

To Joann Davis, for the idea for this project

To Colleen Kaplin, for your effervescent spirit and your relentless attention to detail

To Julia Kushnirsky and Jackie Merri Meyer, for the love and care in handling the artwork

To Durba Ghosh, master coordinator, for being the glue that holds this project together

To Larry Kirshbaum, Nanscy Neiman, and Ellen Herrick, for your continual enthusiasm and support

To Pam Bernstein, my agent at William Morris, for your careful handling of this project

To Joe and Betty Weider, for inventing and promoting the training principles used in this book and by the champions, and for your wonderful magazines: **Muscle and Fitness, Shape, Men's Fitness,** and **Flex**

To Don Banks, for your creative, relentless attention to perfect photography

To Jodi Pollutro, for your creative sensitivity working with hair and makeup

To Augustine, Larry, Robert, Vito, and Dave, the "before" and "after" men in Chapter 2, for daring to believe that with persistence, changes can be made

To family and friends, for your continual love and support

Contents

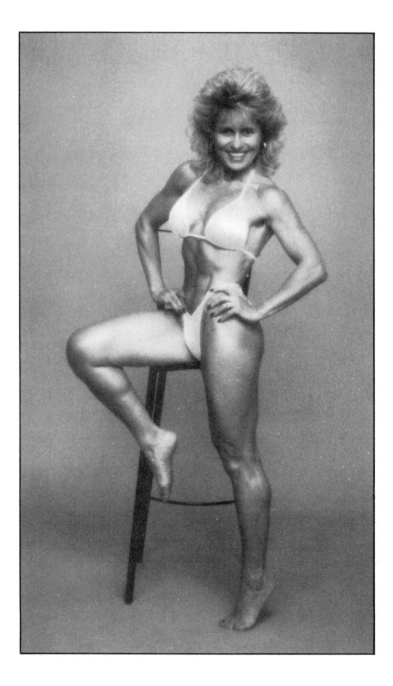

Introduction

Several years ago, when I was Fitness Director at the Aspen Club in Aspen, Colorado, I discovered the training techniques of Joyce Vedral, spelled out in her books *Now or Never* and *Hard Bodies*. Being a continuing student in the fitness industry, I applied her methods to myself and to my clients, and discovered the result was a transformation of virtually any "body" in a matter of weeks. Since that time, I have been using her techniques, in combination with my own, to train celebrities, business executives, professional athletes, and people ranging in fitness level from beginner to most advanced. The results have been excellent.

I've also used these principles in my work as Spa Director at Canyon Ranch in Arizona, and I use them now as Spa and Fitness Director at Cal-A-Vie Health Spa (identified by *Lifestyles of the Rich and Famous* as the Number Two spa in the world) in Vista, California.

I must confess that the first time I picked up one of Joyce Vedral's books I was a bit skeptical. "Can a woman really know how men should train?" I asked myself. But after examining her techniques, I quickly realized that Joyce had taken the secrets of champion male bodybuilders and translated them into a modified program suitable for the average person, male or female.

Since that time, I have used her methods in working with everyone who wants to achieve top fitness in the minimum of time. I have worked with professional tennis players (Martina Navratilova and Chris Evert), a professional hockey team (the New Jersey Devils), and a professional baseball team (the Houston Astros). I've also worked with triathletes, runners, professional skiers, and a number of celebrities, among them Paula Abdul, Kathy Smith, Jane Fonda, and Don Henley. I have also worked with many busy executives who want to look and feel their best without spending all day at it.

What has most impressed me about Joyce's techniques are their power to achieve the goal in a limited time. Her methods are to-the-point. They get the job done. What's more, those who use them do not become "muscle bound."

It has been my experience that the Number One area of concern to men who are not seeking to be bodybuilders is the stomach or abdominal area. Time and again, I have been asked to show men how to flatten their stomachs and get "rips" (add definition) in that area. The following pages will show you the method I've used to transform my own abdominal area, and that of hundreds of men and women from all walks of life whom I have trained.

While it is true that I've served as personal trainer to many clients who enjoyed and could afford the one-to-one attention of a professional athlete, I can say wholeheartedly that no personal trainer is needed to help you achieve the results described in this book. In typical Joyce Vedral style, the exercise descriptions and the photographs are crystal clear. In fact, the "before" and "after" photographs you'll see depict men who got in shape by following the techniques and instructions in this book, just as you will.

Chances are you've attended "abs" classes or tried other methods of getting your stomach in shape—methods that have failed. I believe this book provides the missing link to your program. It spells out a sure-fire way to get dramatic results in twelve weeks time. In fact, I believe that if you follow the plan exactly as it is laid out, you will find it virtually impossible not to be thrilled with your progress.

A further note: There's good news for you men who are extremely out of shape. The more out of shape you are, the more dramatic your progress will be! Just take a look at the "before" and "after" men in Chapter 2 if you need to be convinced.

So let's get on with the program. If you begin now, in three months time you'll have a whole new outlook, especially when you look down—because your "gut" will no longer obscure your view.

— Kent Maurer

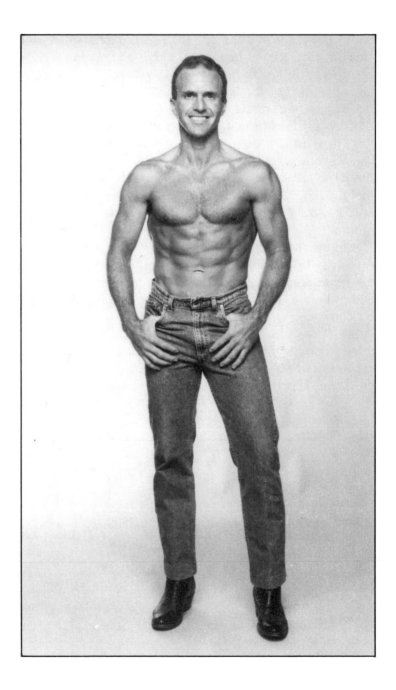

1

"I JUST WANT TO GET RID OF MY GUT"

I don't want to look like a bodybuilder. I just want to get rid of this gut." These familiar words have been spoken by men all over the country. Most men are not interested in looking like Arnold Schwarzenegger. In fact, many men do not really care to increase the size of their chests or biceps, or to broaden their backs. "I don't want to have to buy new suits," they say. "Just give me a workout that will get rid of this paunch."

This book is an answer to their call. It lays out a no-nonsense plan that gets right to the root of the problem—a plan that will get you to your goal in just twelve weeks time. It is based on the technique of muscle isolation, first used by bodybuilders.

For example, suppose a bodybuilder looks great in every way, except he has small, insignificant calves. In order to bring that body part up to par, he must exercise his calves in isolation of all other body parts, until his calves are developed and shaped appropriately.

Sometimes it is not the calves that are the problem, but the chest, or the shoulders, or the back. And sometimes it is the abdominals ("gut") that need special work. Bodybuilders have learned how to change any body part, in isolation from other body parts, in order to shape that part into perfect form. This book applies their secrets to the one body part that concerns most men—the abdominal muscles.

YOU CAN GET RID OF YOUR GUT, BUT...

As you exercise your abdominal muscles according to this workout, those muscles will grow stronger. However, if you are carrying additional body fat, chances are that fat will be stored in your abdominal area, and cover your developing muscles. In fact, the favorite place for male storage of excess body fat is the stomach. Think about that for a moment: You rarely see a man with fat arms or legs. It's always the "rubber tire" around his midsection that seems to hold the fat.

What does all of this mean? You can train your abdominal muscles correctly and develop a steely girdle of perfect muscles in that area, but unless you also get rid of your excess body fat, no one, not even you, will see those muscles. True, you will be able to feel them if you pound on your stomach. It will be clear that under the fat, there is a hardness that wasn't there before. But you won't be able to see what you've worked to accomplish until you lose that ten, fifteen, twenty, or more pounds of "blubber" that is covering your muscles.

In order to get rid of the excess fat covering your developing muscles, you will have to follow a low-fat eating plan. It's not a "diet" in the traditional sense of the word—a temporary plan to lose weight. It is a new way of eating—for life—a low-fat way of eating. (See Chapter 5 for details.)

FIFTEEN MINUTES OF EXERCISE A DAY WILL DO IT

In just a few minutes, I'll outline my gut-busting program in detail, but for now let me spell out for you what you can expect if you are willing to invest fifteen minutes, four to six days a week: a brand-new stomach in less than three months. And you'll see and feel an incredible difference in a matter of weeks.

How can this be? Is it possible to reshape a body part in such a short time period? Actually, fifteen minutes is a lot of exercise time to devote to just one body part. In fact, champion bodybuilders devote just that amount of time—or less—to their stomachs. Bodybuilders train nine body parts, not just one. They train three to five body parts per session, and devote about twenty to thirty minutes to each body part. Since you are training only your stomach, you will only have to devote fifteen minutes in all to your exercise program.

But if you are not a bodybuilder, why do you have to devote even fifteen minutes to your stomach? Why not five or ten minutes? True, you would get excellent results even if you did a mere half of the exercises prescribed in this book. (In fact, the men in the next chapter only did four of the seven exercises.) But your goal is to see dramatic results. You are sick and tired of your unsightly stomach. Why not say, "Bombs away!" and go the extra mile? This program will give you a top-rate stomach, one that will be the envy of males everywhere. What's more, it will get you to your goal quickly, and that's what you want.

Later, when you see how great your stomach looks, you'll probably want to exercise the rest of your body. You'll only have to invest ten to fifteen minutes per body part, and exercise those body parts every other day. The whole daily program will take about thirty to forty minutes. But for now, since all you want is a gorgeous stomach, forget the rest of your body and find out what you can do by challenging your stomach muscles only.

THE SYSTEM IS FOOL-PROOF

Chances are you've seen other books on abdominal training for men. Most of these books are written by well-meaning sports figures, models, movie stars, or the like. The routines prescribed in them are partially effective, and based upon the experience of the writer. This book, on the other hand, is written by an author who has worked with the ultimate experts in body shaping—champion bodybuilders, who knows all the secrets of transforming the body in the quickest, most effective way possible.

The fact is, sports figures, models, and movie stars come to me, an expert in bodybuilding and body shaping, after observing that their time-consuming programs produce little or no results. They know that when you have a toothache, you go to a dentist, not a foot doctor. When you have trouble with your car, you bring it to a mechanic, not to a furniture repair shop. And when you have a problem shaping a body part, you bring it to a "body-building expert," not to someone who just looks good or claims to be a fitness expert. There are many fitness experts who can tell you how to build overall stamina, a healthy heart and lungs, how to be flexible, and so on. But they cannot tell you with on-the-dime specificity how to get the ideal stomach in the least amount of time.

So you've come to the right place to get the job done. Now let's get it done.

WHAT IS INVOLVED IN THIS PROGRAM

You will do seven exercises for your abdominal muscles. After a gentle break-in period that will last only as long as you need it, you will be performing three sets of fifteen to twenty-five repetitions of each exercise—twenty-one sets in all. (A simple explanation of terms is provided in Chapter 3.) In other words, it's "bombs away" on your abdominal area. Your developing muscles will replace the fat that presently inhabits that area (assuming, of course, that you follow the low-fat eating plan).

The Magic Seven

There are seven basic exercises in this program:

Sit-ups	V-ups
Crunches	Serratus pulls
Leg raises	Oblique crunches
Knee-ins	

The exercises cover the three areas of the stomach: the upper abdominal area, the lower abdominal area, and the side abdominal area. Substitutes are provided for those who cannot perform certain exercises. (For a detailed description of the abdominal muscles, see Chapter 3.)

WHY OTHER PROGRAMS FAIL

Muscles must be handled with care. They are in some sense like plants. More is not always better. For example, too much water can drown a plant. In the same way, too many repetitions can erode a muscle. A good example of this type of overtraining can be seen in most "abs" classes, where well-meaning fitness instructors have clients over-train abdominal muscles for thirty minutes, doing high repetitions. All that accomplishes is the wearing away of hard-earned abdominal muscle.

Other abdominal programs fail because they provide too little concentration on the abdominal muscles. Circuit training is an example of this. The exerciser is asked to do only one or two exercises for each body part before moving on to the next body part, with abdominals treated like the rest. There is not enough concentration on each muscle group in isolation of others. You see, in order to develop, a muscle must be forced literally to rise to the occasion by concentrated demand. Circuit training does not provide enough concentrated effort on your abdominal area to get results.

WHY SPORTS CAN NEVER GET YOUR ABDOMINALS IN SHAPE

Did you ever see a marathon runner with a little paunch? It's quite common. And many a tennis player is sporting a spare tire. How many golfers, racquetball players, squash players, swimmers, and even wrestlers are carrying excess baggage in the stomach department? Quite a few. If sports were able to get rid of the gut, why would these men, some of them champions, still have less than ideal midsections?

WHY THIS PROGRAM IS SUPERIOR TO OTHER ABDOMINAL PROGRAMS

This program stands alone, in that it is based upon time-tested principles of champion bodybuilders. It utilizes the principles of muscle isolation and peak contraction, dynamic tension and continual pressure. It ensures that you do not overtrain, as do well-meaning athletes who foolishly brag, "I did five hundred sit-ups this morning. It ensures that you do not undertrain, like those who rely on circuit training or sports to reshape their stomachs. This program provides just the right amount of challenge to get the job done in the quickest, most efficient way possible.

I have trained with champions for years. I will show you how to exercise the way the champions do, using no more than three sets of fifteen to twenty-five repetitions per exercise, and no more than twenty-one sets of exercise for your abdominal workout.

THE PROMISE

If you follow this program as instructed, it will be literally impossible not to see results in three months time. You will be the envy of your friends. (See the "before" and "after" pictures in Chapter 2.) You, too, can become an "after." Take a photograph of yourself before you start the workout. Then three months later, take another photograph. I would love to see the result. (You can send it to me at the P.O. box listed at the end of Chapter 7.)

WHAT ABOUT THE WOMEN?

Yes. Women can use this program. In fact, if there's a woman in your life and you'd like to work out with her, consider the "partnering" workout described in Chapter 7. When it comes to abdominals, the exercises for men and women are basically the same, only where weight is suggested, women use lighter weights than men.

THIS IS A HOME WORKOUT, BUT YOU CAN DO IT IN THE GYM

You need no equipment to do this workout. It can be done at home in any room. If you decide to use weights, all you have to do is purchase one or two hand-held weights, but that will not be necessary for at least a month or two.

If you choose to do the workout in a gym, follow the gym alternatives. However, keep in mind that most champion bodybuilders rarely use machines in their abdominal workouts. They choose, for the most part, to ignore the machines, because they know that when it comes to abdominals, machines are second-best to working solo with no weights or light weights.

However, if you love the abdominal machines and want to substitute them for some of the exercises here when you go to the gym, that's all right. I've indicated names of the machines you can use for a substitute. Don't worry—you'll still see major development. Just not as much as if you followed the program exactly—without the use of machines.

WHAT YOU WILL GET FROM THIS WORKOUT AND EATING PLAN

1. Reduced overall body fat, expecially around the "middle"
2. A strong, well-defined, muscular stomach in twelve weeks time
3. Increased overall strength (because the stomach is the center of strength)
4. More energy
5. Increased self-esteem
6. Lower cholesterol level

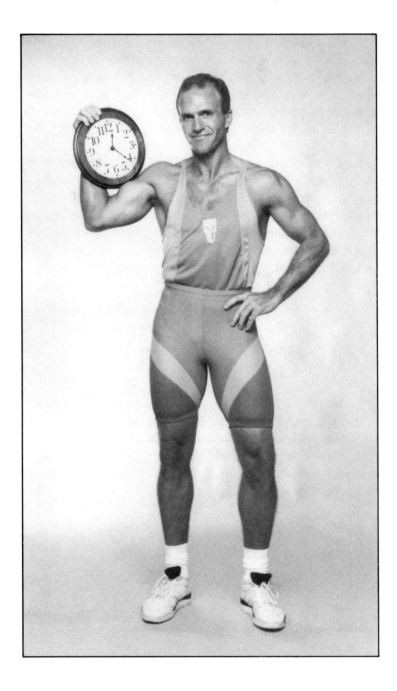

2

HOW LONG WILL IT TAKE?

Your progress will depend upon the shape you're in now. But no matter what shape you're in, you will see major results in twelve weeks time—or in nine to eighteen hours of workout time (three to six fifteen-minute workout sessions per week).

Does three months seem like a long time? Think of it this way: In three months, you'll either be in the same shape you're in now, in worse shape, or in better shape. And chances are, if you do nothing you'll be in worse shape. This is especially true if you've passed the age of thirty.

You see, every year after thirty, unless you do something to reverse it, muscles atrophy a small amount. Along with muscle atrophy, comes accumulation of fat. This is due to the fact that muscle tissue is the only body material that is active. The more muscle tissue on your body, the higher your metabolism. As you age, if you do nothing to replace the atrophying muscle, your metabolism slows down. When this happens, you gain weight, or, to put it bluntly, get fat—even though you are eating the same amount of food you ate before, and are doing the same amount of exercise.

All is not lost. You can recover the muscle you are losing—and then some. As this is an abdominal workout, you will recover lost abdominal muscle and add new muscles in that area in the bargain. Later, if you are convinced that this program has made a difference, you may decide to work on the rest of your body. (See the bibliography for references to *The Fat-Burning Workout* or *Now or Never.*

THE RIGHT WEIGHT BUT YOU STILL HAVE A GUT

If you are a man who looks great in clothing, not really overweight but carrying a little "paunch" that just seems to get in the way, you fall into this category. With the gut buster program you will be in ideal abdominal shape in three months time. (See our "before" and "after" photographs of Augustine and Larry.)

After using the program for three weeks, you will begin to feel a lot stronger. Why is this so, when you are exercising only the stomach area? It's because the stomach is the center of strength, or, in martial arts parlance, the "hara"—the seat of all energy. In short, the stronger your stomach muscles, the more powerful your basic energy thrust.

In addition to feeling an increase in strength, you will begin to see a change in the shape and quality of your stomach. It will be reduced in size, as excess fat gives up its post. You will also see fine lines of definition beginning to show along your side abdominals (obliques). There will be some definition beginning to show on your upper abdominal area.

In six weeks, you'll see further reduction of your "gut" size, and in addition you'll notice more definition in your upper abdominal area. Perhaps to your amazement, you'll also begin to see a change in your lower stomach. The little "belly" will be reduced in size, and some definition will be evident in that area.

AUGUSTINE

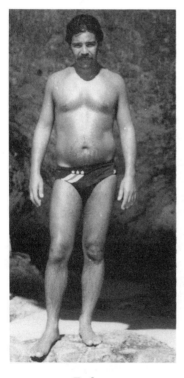 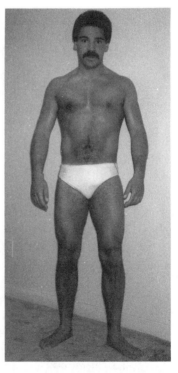

Before   **After**

LARRY

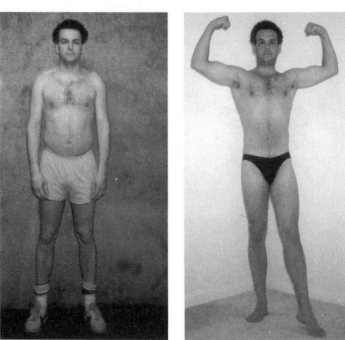

Before   After

In three months, you will have a near-perfect abdominal area. Why do we say near-perfect? The answer is simple: Although you won't be able to imagine that your stomach could improve still further, it will. As you continue to work out, your abdominal area will get harder and harder, and become more and more well defined.

Two of the men in this book fall into this category: Augustine and Larry. Neither man was significantly overweight when he began this program, yet both had little "paunches" that they couldn't seem to get rid of no matter what they did. Look at their "before" and "after" pictures, summarizing graphically the results after three months. As time goes on, these men will see further improvement.

UP TO THIRTY POUNDS OVERWEIGHT WITH A LARGE PAUNCH

If you carry around an excess of weight, there's good news for you gentlemen, too. Even though you will not reach your ideal goal in three months, you will realize it is in reach (see the "before" and "after" pictures that follow of Robert, Vito, and Dave).

In three weeks time, you will feel a lot stronger, and assuming you are following the low-fat eating plan, you will see a significant reduction in the size of your gut. You will not see definition yet, because there is probably still too much fat covering your abdominal muscles.

In six weeks you will notice that your stomach size is greatly reduced, with some definition in your obliques (side abdominal area) and in your upper abdominal area.

In nine weeks your lower abdominal area will show a greater reduction, and you will see further definition in your upper abdominal area and your obliques. You may begin to see some slight definition in your lower abdominal area. In three months, you will see significant progress in your entire abdominal area.

Notice the three men in the "before" and "after" section of this book. Robert was twenty pounds overweight. Three months later, he is only five pounds overweight, and well on his way to perfect abdominals. He doesn't have much definition yet, because there's still a layer of fat covering his stomach, but in another month, as he follows the

ROBERT

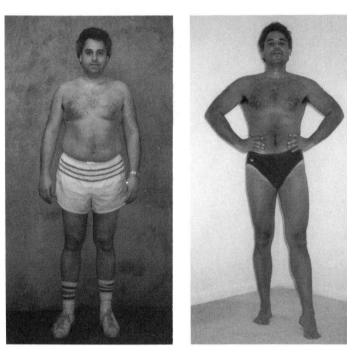

Before   **After**

low-fat eating plan and continues to do the workout, his stomach will be "ripped."

Vito is twenty-five pounds overweight in his "before" photograph. Three months later, he is only five pounds overweight. But it isn't his weight loss that has caused the entire change in his abdominal area. He's been working diligently five times a week, and as you can see, he now has definition in his upper abdominals and his obliques. He can now also "flex" his stomach to show off his progress. Before, he could have flexed away, and no muscle would show, because his stomach was still covered with a mountain of fat.

When looking at the photographs, you will probably say to yourself, "Vito looks as if he's made the most progress of all the men. He appeared the worst in the beginning, and now he looks the best." Vito is a classic case of the man we discussed in Chapter 1—the man who carries nearly all of his excess fat in his abdominal area. That's why he looks nearly perfect now.

VITO

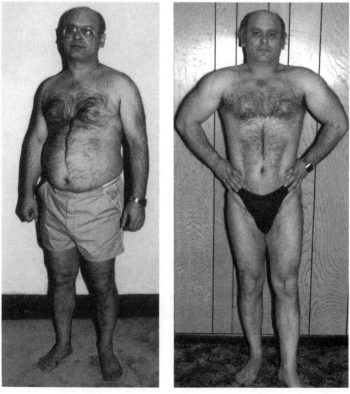

Before   **After**

DAVE

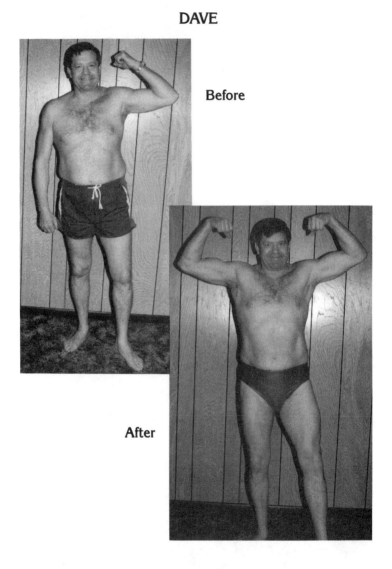

Before

After

Now look at Dave. He was thirty pounds overweight to begin with, and he is ten pounds overweight now. Some of that excess weight is lying on his developing abdominals in the form of fat. But if you look closely, you can see that much of the fat has been eliminated from his abdominal area, and you can see definition in his upper abdominal area and his obliques. Why does it seem as if Vito has made so much more progress than Dave? Dave's case points out a simple truth, one we all know: Everyone is different genetically. While most men carry the bulk of their fat in the abdominal area, some have excess fat more evenly distributed over their bodies. Dave has apparently lost fat more evenly all over his body—from his back, his shoulders, his arms, etc.

In addition, Dave is still ten pounds overweight. He will continue to lose his excess fat, and in three to five months will have near-perfect abdominals.

MORE THAN THIRTY POUNDS OVERWEIGHT

If you fall into this category, don't despair. You will surprise yourself by the rapid progress you will make. It will just take you a little longer to get to your goal. Allow a month for every five to seven pounds overweight to goal time. You will see progress all along the way, but remember one thing: You must follow the low-fat eating plan, and you must follow the abdominal workout religiously. There is no room for compromise. If you want the payment, you have to do the work. It's that simple.

Fortunately for you, there seems to be a strange advantage when it comes to progress if you've seriously neglected your muscles. The human body is a survival system. It "knows" that strong, well-developed muscles are necessary to help you survive day to day. So when you finally begin to challenge previously neglected muscles, they cooperate 100 percent; they seem to "leap" into shape. The fact of it is: Your body wants to get in shape and will help you along.

WHAT ABOUT AGE?

There's good news for men under thirty, and great news for men over thirty. For younger men, you will see even more rapid progress than is described above. All of the men in the "before" and "after" pictures are over thirty—they range from thirty-three to fifty-two. (Augustine is thirty-three, Larry is thirty-five, Robert is thirty-six, Vito is forty-five, and Dave is fifty-two.) If you are under thirty, you will probably progress even faster than these men, who must also make up for the muscle atrophy that takes place after thirty.

If you are over thirty, take your inspiration from the men in this chapter. You will surprise yourself as to the rapid progress you make. What's more, along with looking younger, you'll feel younger, too, because as previously atrophying muscles are replaced, and then increased, your body will actually have gotten younger—muscle-wise.

True, your younger compatriots may progress a little faster, but that is only because they do not have to make up for the slight muscle atrophy that takes place every year after thirty. If you work hard, you can more than make up the difference. In fact, it's been our experience that men over thirty make the best progress. Perhaps this is due to the fact that they realize they can no longer rely upon the natural physique of youth to get them through!

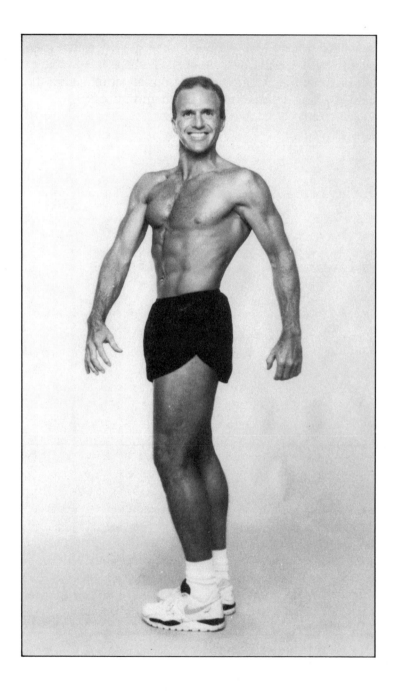

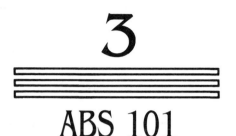

ABS 101

In order to get the most out of this workout, it's a good idea to learn a little about the physiology of the abdominal area. That will give you a clear picture of your stomach muscles. Then as you work out, you can visualize these muscles getting stronger. In fact, you can learn to "tell" your muscles to develop as you exercise.

Before you begin your workout, you'll need to become familiar with some basic exercise expressions, such as "repetition," "set," "muscle isolation," "peak contraction," etc. You will also want information as to why the abdominal muscles are trained differently than are other muscle groups, even though at this point you may not be planning to exercise any muscles other than your abdominals.

THE ABDOMINAL MUSCLES

Your stomach or "gut" is actually the combination of four muscle groups: the rectus abdominis, the external obliques, the internal obliques, and the transversus abdominis. For exercise purposes, however, we divide the abdominal area into three groups: the upper abdominals, the lower abdominals, and the side abdominals.

The rectus abdominus covers the upper and lower abdominal areas, and is really one long segmented muscle. However, exercises for this muscle are commonly divided into "upper" and "lower" abdominals, because it is difficult to find one exercise that places equal stress on both areas of this muscle at the same time. You will note which area of the abdominals is emphasized as you read the exercise instructions.

The rectus abdominis is attached to the fifth through seventh ribs, near the breastbone, and runs along the abdominal wall. It is attached on the other end to the pubic bone of the pelvis. This muscle functions to pull the torso toward the lower body when sitting up from a supine (lying on your back) position.

The external oblique muscles originate at the side of the lower ribs, and run diagonally to the rectus abdominis. These muscles are attached to the sheath of fibrous tissue that surrounds the rectus abdominis. The external oblique muscles, together with the internal oblique muscles, comprise what we call the "side abdominal area."

The external oblique muscles work with other muscles to rotate the trunk and flex the torso. It is the external oblique muscles, when well developed, that provide definition in the side abdominal area and help to make your waist look smaller.

The internal oblique muscles lie beneath the external

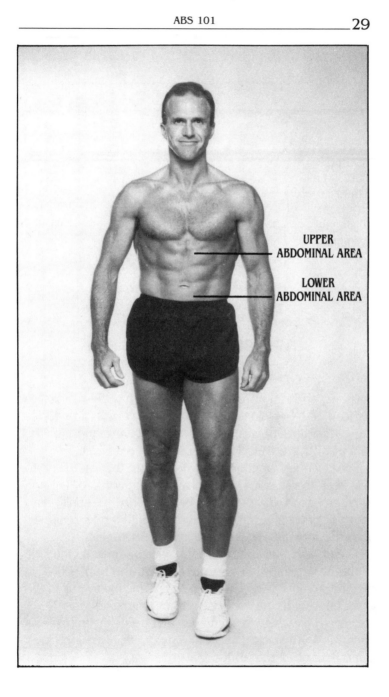

UPPER
ABDOMINAL AREA

LOWER
ABDOMINAL AREA

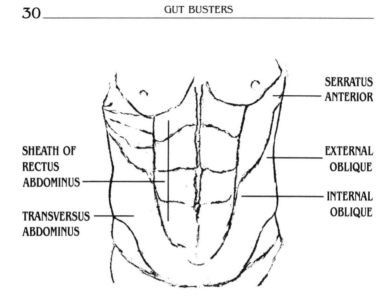

SERRATUS ANTERIOR

SHEATH OF RECTUS ABDOMINUS

TRANSVERSUS ABDOMINUS

EXTERNAL OBLIQUE

INTERNAL OBLIQUE

THE ABDOMINAL MUSCLES

obliques, and run at roughly right angles to them. It is this angle that determines the size of one's waistline (once excess fat disappears). The more acute the angle of the joining of these muscles, the narrower the waist.

The obliques function to twist and turn the torso, and to help keep the waistline area from slumping forward. Twisting motions, such as provided by the "oblique pull" and "oblique crunch" exercises, help to define and strengthen both the internal and external oblique muscles.

The transversus abdominis muscles originate at the side of the abdominal wall and travel along the midsection of the abdominal cavity. These muscles function to pull in the lower stomach. All exercises that emphasize the lower abdominal area help to strengthen and define the transversus abdominis muscles. (See our anatomy illustration for a clear view of all the abdominal muscles.)

EXERCISE TERMS

The exercise terms here are given in order of magnitude. We start with the all-encompassing term "routine," which covers all exercises, then go to "exercise" and break that down to its components, "sets." We then break sets down into yet smaller components, "repetitions." Rests are described last.

Routine. All of the exercises performed for a given body part. For example, this is your abdominal routine, and it consists of seven exercises.

Exercise. The designated movement performed to strengthen a given body part. For example, this routine contains the following exercises: sit-ups, crunches, V-ups, leg raises, knee-ins, oblique pulls, and oblique crunches.

Set. A specified number of movements (repetitions) to be performed without resting. In this routine, each set will consist of fifteen to twenty-five repetitions.

Repetition, or "rep." The complete movement of a given exercise, from starting point to midpoint and back to starting point again. For example, one repetition of the crunch involves raising the shoulders off the ground (on the ground is start position) to as high as possible (midpoint position) then back to flat on the ground (start position).

Rest. A brief pause between sets. In this routine, you will rest thirty to sixty seconds between sets.

MUSCLE ACTION TERMS

Flex. To contract the muscle. For example, when you curl into the midpoint of the crunch (your shoulders are off the ground), your upper abdominal muscles will be in the flexed position. In order to make maximum progress, we advise you to cooperate with this flexed position by squeezing your muscles as hard as possible. When you do this, you will achieve "peak contraction." You will continually be reminded to do this in the exercise instructions.

Peak contraction. Complete and total contraction of the muscle—a step beyond flexing. For example, when in the shoulders-off-the-floor position of a crunch, the upper abdominal muscles are in the contracted, or "flexed," state. At this point, if you exert additional effort, squeezing the upper abdominals as hard as possible, you achieve peak contraction.

Stretch. The stretch position is the opposite of the flex position. The muscle is elongated rather than shortened. For example, in performing the crunch, your abdominal muscles are in the stretch position when your shoulders are flat to the ground.

MUSCLE APPEARANCE

Muscle Mass. Mass in this context refers to the actual size of a given muscle. Abdominal muscles are smaller in mass than are any of the other eight body parts: chest, shoulders, biceps, triceps, thighs, back, gluteus maximus, and calves. For this reason, they require less weight and higher repetitions for optimum development.

Muscularity. This refers to the amount of muscle in given parts of the body, as opposed to fatty tissue. For example, when you start this workout, your abdominal muscles will have little muscularity (there will be lots of fat surrounding your abdominal muscles). As you continue to follow this routine, and observe the low-fat eating plan, your abdominal muscles will increase, while the fat in that area decreases. You will have a high degree of muscularity in your abdominal area.

Definition. The clear delineation and visibility of a muscle. Definition can be seen only after muscularity is achieved. All excess fat must be removed from the muscle before significant definition is visible. Your abdominals will slowly begin to show definition as you follow the routine and eating plan. After you have been following the routine for three months, and if by then you are not carrying more than five pounds of excess fat, you will see a good deal of definition in your abdominal area.

EXERCISE EQUIPMENT

Dumbbell. A short metal bar that can be held in one hand. A dumbbell has raised, rounded ends that are usually permanently fixed to the bar. You may use a dumbbell held between your feet for some of the abdominal exercises in this workout.

Plate. A plate is a disc-shaped weight that is usually placed on either side of a barbell. For our purposes, a plate weighing from ten to twenty-five pounds can be held on the abdominal area as you perform certain exercises. Dumbbells and plates can be purchased in any sporting goods store, or you may order them through the P.O. box given on page 102.

GENERAL EXERCISE PRINCIPLES

Muscle isolation. The method of exercising each body part independently of other body parts, until that part has been challenged into significant growth and development. In order to ensure maximum growth, development, and strengthening of a given body part, you must provide that body part with uninterrupted work. In short, you achieve nothing doing one or two sets of abdominal exercises, then one or two sets of another exercise, and then skip back to an exercise for the abdominals. You must perform a minimum number of sets on a body part with only short rest periods (from thirty to sixty seconds) or little or no development will take place.

Intensity. This refers to the degree of difficulty of the exercises performed. Intensity can be increased by adding to the number of repetitions, increasing the weight load, increasing the number of sets, or reducing the rest periods between sets. Your abdominal workout is very intense, because you are doing the maximum number of sets allowed for the abdominal area—twenty-one. You can regulate the intensity of your workout, however, by deciding whether to do the minimum of fifteen repetitions per set, or the maximum of twenty-five repetitions per set.

Dynamic tension. The application of pressure on a muscle in the stretching or elongating stage of an exercise movement. For example, when performing the crunch, if you exert tension on the upper abdominal muscles as you lower yourself to the floor, you are applying "dynamic tension."

Continual tension. The constant application of tension or pressure on the working muscle, both on the flexing aspect of the movement, and on the stretching aspect of the movement. For example, if you exert continual flexing pressure on the upper abdominal muscles as you raise your shoulders off the ground, and continue to apply pressure on the upper abdominals as you lower yourself to the ground, you are applying the principle of continual tension. In other words, constant peak contraction plus constant dynamic tension equals continual tension. If you apply continual tension on your abdominal muscles as you exercise, you will get hard, well-defined muscles. You can greatly speed up your progress by applying this principle.

HOW DO ABDOMINAL EXERCISES DIFFER FROM ALL OTHER EXERCISES?

For exercise purposes, there are eight basic body parts on men: chest, shoulders, triceps, biceps, back, thighs, calves, and abdominals. (Women have an additional body part to exercise, the buttocks. Men do not exercise the buttocks independently of quadriceps or thighs, because of their physiology.) Of the eight, the only one that is not exercised with significant weight is the abdominal area. For example, you may do a bench press with one hundred pounds. You may do a shoulder press of seventy pounds, or a triceps pushdown of a hundred pounds, and so on. But you would never use more than a twenty-five pound plate when doing a sit-up (and most men would use less weight—or no weight).

Another difference between abdominals and other body parts is the number of repetitions. Other body parts are exercised with six to fifteen repetitions per set, depending upon the heaviness of the weight used. Never do people who know what they're doing go higher than fifteen repetitions for any body part other than the abdominals (except for women who want to reduce their thighs and buttocks).

To go higher than fifteen repetitions for other body parts would be to wear away the muscle. Abdominals are different. Because they are small muscles to begin with, and need strengthening and defining rather than increased size, higher repetitions and lower weights are required. In general, the maximum number of repetitions per set for abdominals is twenty-five. Once in a while, it is okay to do sets of fifty repetitions, just to test your strength.

MUSCLE SORENESS

Muscle soreness is the result of microscopic tears in the fibers of the ligaments and tendons connecting the muscles, with slight internal swelling accompanying those tears. Soreness is quite normal for the first week or two after starting a vigorous workout program—even if you do break in gently. The minuscule tears suffered are in fact necessary if you're to make any progress in strengthening and developing your abdominal muscles.

If you feel sore the day after working out, be happy. Know that your previously dormant muscles are now being forced to come to life. Whatever you do, don't stop working out just because you are sore. Work right through the soreness. In fact, you will feel better immediately after the workout, because the workout serves as a gentle massage to your aching muscles.

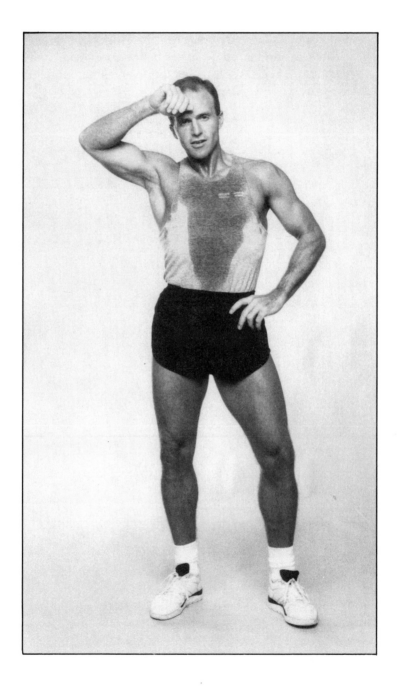

4

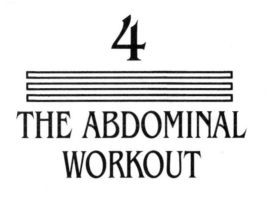

THE ABDOMINAL WORKOUT

There are seven abdominal exercises in this workout. We have no intention of babying you. You will do each and every exercise on each workout day, or you will do the substitute. However, if you are extremely out of shape, and/or you have never worked out before, or you want to take it slow, we do have a "break in gently" plan. That allows you to do less repetitions of these exercises in the beginning, so that you can achieve full power gradually.

Some of you have worked out before, and are in fact in great physical condition. You can try the full program and see how you fare. If you are able to perform the entire routine with little problem, great. Why waste time with the break-in program? On the other hand, it's important that you be honest with yourself. If you try the full program and find that it's too much for you, cut back to one of the break-in-gently plans. It's better to go slowly and eventually arrive at the goal, than to go too quickly and quit in disgust!

HOW MANY DAYS A WEEK SHOULD YOU WORK OUT?

Ideally, you should exercise your abdominal muscles five to six days a week until you reach your goal, then three to four days a week after that. In other words, for the first three months, you should work very hard. After that, if you are at goal, you can cut back to a maintenance program of three to four days a week. However, if you have time to do only three sessions per week, you will still see a major change take place in your stomach area in a matter of months. The change will not take place as quickly, nor will it be as dramatic as it would be had you worked the extra two or three days.

WHAT YOU WILL DO EACH WORKOUT DAY

You will do three sets of fifteen-to-twenty-five repetitions of each exercise. Never do more than twenty-five repetitions. Since you will be doing seven exercises, you will be doing twenty-one sets for your abdominals in all. Do not do any more sets than that, or you will wear away hard-earned muscle.

WHAT ABOUT WEIGHTS?

In order to build a strong steely belt of muscle across your abdominal area, you will have to use relatively light weights for certain exercises. No matter how strong you are, however, never use weights higher than those suggested in the exercise instructions. If you do, at worst you will injure your back; at best you will reduce the efficacy of your abdominal routine. That's because you will force other muscles to come into play in order to "help" your abdominal muscles cope with an otherwise impossible amount of work.

RESTING BETWEEN SETS

You will rest thirty to sixty seconds between sets. After a few months, you may find yourself wanting to jump into the next set after ten or fifteen seconds. You can do that. Listen to your body. If your body tells you to go ahead, just do it. However, if your body tells you to rest more than sixty seconds, say "No." You've got to push your body forward. If you can't do the next set after sixty seconds, temporarily reduce your repetitions and gradually work your way up again.

WHEN TO EXERCISE

It's a good idea to get your abdominal routine out of the way in the morning. If you do it at the crack of dawn, it's out of the way. What's more, it's a great way to start the day. It gives you a feeling of accomplishment, and in addition, it helps to speed up your metabolism for hours after, giving you early morning mental and physical energy.

However, if you are more comfortable with an afternoon or evening session, there is no reason why you can't do it then. However, it's better to avoid working out right before bedtime. Allow at least an hour and a half after working out to wind down. Your speedy metabolism may keep you awake otherwise.

BREAK-IN PLAN FOR THOSE WHO ARE ONLY SLIGHTLY OUT OF SHAPE

Instead of doing all three sets of each exercise for fifteen-to-twenty-five repetitions, do three sets in the following progression. Use no weights, regardless of exercise instructions. (Rest a full sixty seconds between sets if necessary).

Week 1.   3 sets of 5 to 7 repetitions
Week 2.   3 sets of 8 to 10 repetitions
Week 3.   3 sets of 11 to 15 repetitions
Week 4.   3 sets of 15 to 25 repetitions

After the fourth week, you may begin using the weights as prescribed in specific exercise instructions.

BREAK-IN PLAN FOR THOSE WHO HAVE NEVER EXERCISED BEFORE AND/OR ARE BADLY OUT OF SHAPE

Instead of doing all three sets of each exercise for fifteen-to-twenty-five repetitions, do three sets of the following progression. Use no weights, regardless of exercise instructions. (Rest a full sixty seconds between sets if necessary).

Week 1.   3 sets of 1 to 3 repetitions.
Week 2.   3 sets of 4 to 6 repetitions.
Week 3.   3 sets of 7 to 8 repetitions.
Week 4.   3 sets of 9 to 10 repetitions.
Week 5.   3 sets of 11 to 12 repetitions.
Week 6.   3 sets of 13 to 15 repetitions.
Week 7.   3 sets of 15 or more repetitions.

After week 7, if you wish, you may begin using the weights as described in specific exercise instructions.

THE SIT-UP
Abdominal Exercise #1

Despite the ups and downs of the reputation of the sit-up, it is still one of the most effective exercises to develop your abdominal muscles. However, if your doctor recommends that because of specific back problems, you avoid this exercise, do the alternative. This exercise develops, strengthens, and defines the upper abdominal area (from the waistline to the lower chest area). The lower abdominal area is also strengthened.

Positioning:
Lie flat on your back on the floor, and bend your knees until the soles of your feet are flat on the ground. (You may bend your knees to a lesser extent, and place your ankles under a heavy piece of furniture instead.) Place your hands behind your head.

Exercise:
Using a fluid movement and flexing your entire abdominal area as you work, raise yourself to a sitting position, or until you are nearly perpendicular to the floor. Without resting, and applying continual pressure to your entire abdominal area, return to the start position. Without resting or bouncing off the floor, repeat the movement until you have completed your set.

Tips:
Maintain full control at all times. Beware of the temptation to bounce off the floor or merely rock back and forth. Maintain full attention to flexing your upper and lower abdominal muscles, and keep the pressure on those muscles, even on the

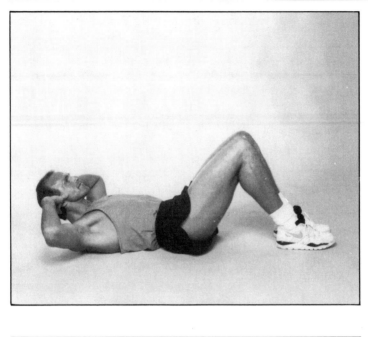

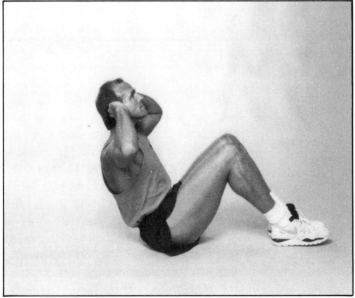

down movement. Remember, in doing these exercises, you will have to fight your own survival system, which will encourage you to invent ways to save your body from work. The goal here is to do *more* work, not less. You must continue to remind your body of that fact.

Gym Alternative:

You may perform this exercise on any gym sit-up machine. You may perform this exercise, according to your ability, on any gym slant board.

Alternative for Sit-up:

See Alternate Crunch.

You may do the advanced slant-board sit-up as shown on page 47. (The slant board is an exercise bench, also featured on page 55. See page 102 for more information about this bench/sit-up board.)

Use of Weights:

You may hold a five-pound weight against your upper abdominal area. You may hold the weight with both hands, or place one hand on the weight, and one hand behind your head as you perform your sit-ups. As you become stronger, you may eventually go as high as a 25-pound weight. Most men prefer to use a disc-shaped weight (plate) wrapped in a towel. However, a dumbbell will serve the purpose just as well. Do not use weights until you can perform three sets of twenty-five repetitions without effort. Then go

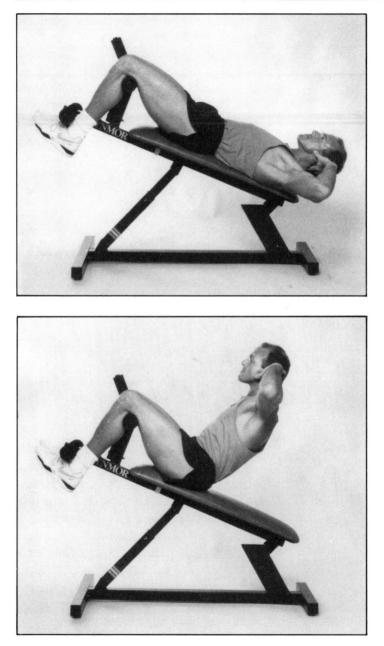

back to fifteen-repetition sets with the lowest weight, and work your way up to twenty-five repetitions again.

Use of ten or more pounds will create thicker abdominal muscles. Kent Maurer, featured on the cover of this book and shown performing the exercises, does not use weights with any exercises. Bodybuilders, who want thicker abdominals, do use them, as do some who are not bodybuilders. The choice is yours.

THE CRUNCH
Abdominal Exercise #2

The crunch develops, strengthens, and defines the upper abdominal area. The lower abdominal area is only slightly affected by this movement.

Positioning: Lie on the floor flat on your back, with your knees bent and feet crossed at the ankles. Place your hands behind your head.

Exercise: Flexing your upper abdominal muscles as hard as possible, slowly raise your shoulders from the floor in a curling movement until your shoulders are completely off the ground. Do *not* raise your back off the ground. Without losing control or dropping to the ground, and continuing to maintain pressure on the upper abdominal muscles, lower yourself to the start position and repeat the movement until you have completed your set.

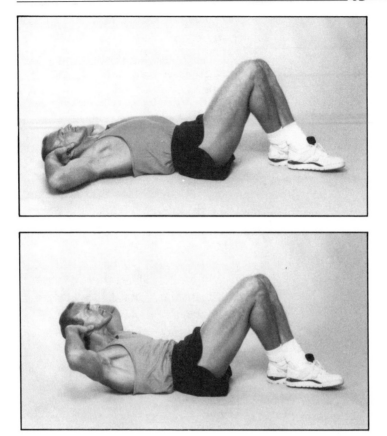

Tips:

Beware of the temptation to lurch off the floor in an effort to gain momentum and make the work easier. Lift from the chest area; do not pull on your neck. As you work, imagine your belly button pressing down through your body into the floor. This will help you to observe good form during the exercise. Breathe naturally.

| Gym Alternative: | You may perform this exercise on any gym crunch machine. If you do use the machine, be sure to observe the above exercise rules of concentration and peak contraction. You do the work, not the machine. |

| Alternative Crunch: | If you are one of those who cannot do sit-ups try this alternative crunch: Do the crunch as described above, only cross your legs at the ankles and raise your knees to chest level and keep them there. Perform the crunch in the same manner as described on page 49. |

| Use of Weights: | Since you are not lifting more than your shoulders off the ground, it is useless to hold weight on your stomach as you perform this movement. To do so would be to waste energy. |

LEG RAISE
Abdominal Exercise #3

This exercise develops, strengthens, and defines the lower abdominal area. It also strengthens the upper abdominal area. If you cannot do leg raises because of medical reasons, do the alternative knee-in.

| Positioning: | Lie on the floor or on a flat exercise bench, and place your hands at your sides. If necessary, you may hold onto the sides of the bench. Bend your legs at the knees to a near L position to take pressure off your back. |

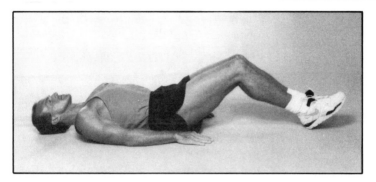

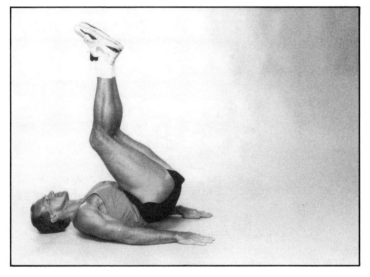

Exercise: Keeping your feet together, raise your
                   legs until they are perpendicular to the
                   floor, flexing your lower abdominal mus-
                   cles as hard as possible throughout the
                   exercise. (If your back hurts, raise your
                   legs higher, to a thigh-to-chest position,
                   as seen in the photograph. This takes
                   pressure off your back.) Without resting,
                   and in full control, return to the start

position, keeping the pressure on your lower abdominal muscles. Repeat the movement until you have completed your set.

Tips:

If you feel stress on your lower back, in addition to raising your legs to a thigh-to-chest position each time, place your hands, palms down, under your buttocks, and keep them there throughout the exercise. Do not allow your legs to just drop back to the start position. Keep your mind riveted on your lower abdominal muscles as you work. Maintain a mental picture of your developing muscles throughout your routine. If you are holding a dumbbell between your feet, keep a firm grip at all times. Do not hold your breath. Breathe naturally.

Gym Alternative:

You may perform this exercise on a flat exercise bench and using a double-looped rope attached to an upper wall pulley machine. Set the weight at twenty pounds and perform your leg raises in the manner described above.

Alternative Leg Raise:

See the alternative knee-in, given with the instructions for Exercise 4.

Use of Weights:

Do not use weights until you can perform three sets of twenty-five repetitions without effort. Then begin with a three-pound weight and go back to fifteen repetitions per set. When you have reached three sets of twenty-five repetitions, you may graduate to five pounds. Never go beyond five pounds for this exercise. That will place undue stress on your back, and will force you to use muscles that are not supposed to be involved in this workout.

KNEE-IN
Abdominal Exercise #4

This exercise develops, strengthens, and defines the lower abdominal area. It also places stress on the upper abdominal area and the external obliques.

Positioning: Sit at the edge of a chair or a flat exercise bench, and hold onto the sides of the chair or bench. Lean back to a 30-degree angle, and extend your legs straight out in front of you.

Exercise: Flexing your lower abdominal muscles as hard as possible and keeping your knees together, pull your knees in toward your chest until you can go no farther. Keeping the tension on your lower abdominal muscles, return to the start position and repeat the movement until you have completed your set.

Tips: Keep your body steady by maintaining a firm grip on the bench. Do not allow yourself to rock back and forth. Focus your mind on your developing lower abdominal muscles. Picture the fat melting away from that area, and hard, well-defined muscles replacing the fat.

Gym Alternative:

You may perform this exercise by sitting at the edge of a flat exercise bench, placed next to a lower wall pulley. Place a double-looped rope around your ankles, and set the weight to twenty pounds. Perform the exercise as above.

Alternative Knee-in:

If you cannot do either the leg raise or the knee-in, you may perform the reverse crunch. Lie flat on the floor with your knees completely bent (to an approximate 90-degree angle). With your knees pointed toward the ceiling, and your hands under your buttocks for support, bring your knees as close to your chest as possible. Return to start position and repeat the movement until you have completed your set.

Use of Weights:

After you have achieved the ability to perform three sets of fifteen repetitions with no weight, you may place a three-pound dumbbell between your ankles. Once you have performed three sets of twenty-five repetitions with that weight, you may advance to five, eight, and then ten pounds. Do *not* go higher than ten pounds or you may injure your back.

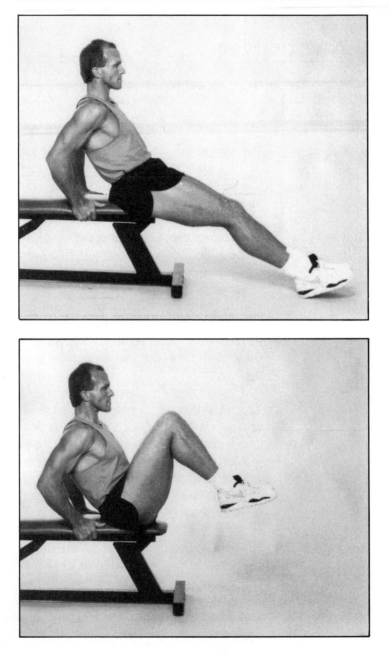

V-UP
Abdominal Exercise #5

This exercise strengthens and develops the upper and lower abdominal areas. It is most challenging. If you cannot perform it, do the alternative V-up.

Positioning: Lie flat on the floor with your legs extended and feet together, keeping your knees slightly bent. Extend your arms straight out behind you.

Exercise: Simultaneously raise your upper and lower body by bringing your arms forward and raising your legs. Keep your legs together as you move. Raise both lower and upper body as high as you can go; then, maintaining complete control, return to the start position. Repeat the movement until you have completed your set.

Tips: This is a difficult exercise. You may be able to do only a few repetitions at first. Don't despair. Do as many as you can without straining. In time your stamina will increase. Remember to flex your upper and lower abdominal area as you work. Maintain full control at all times.

Gym
Alternative: You may perform a modified version of this exercise on the "Roman chair." In this case, you position yourself in the standing "Roman chair" and extend your legs straight out in front of you until they are parallel to the floor. Return to start

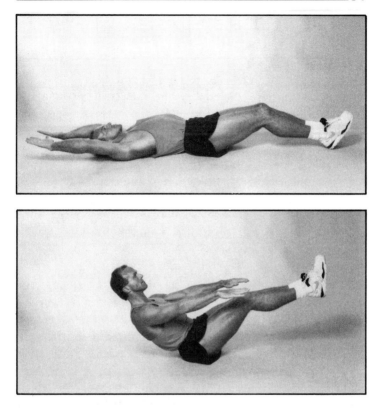

and raise your knees to chest level. Repeat this movement until you have completed your set. (The Roman chair has no seat— only arms and a back, and is high off the ground.)

General Alternative:	Do a combined crunch and lying knee-in. Each crunch–knee-in combination counts as one repetition.
Use of Weights:	No weight is used with this exercise.

THE SERRATUS PULL (For Those "Love Handles")
Abdominal Exercise #6

This exercise strengthens, develops, and defines the oblique muscles. It is called the serratus pull because the initial work begins with the upper side-chest (serratus) muscles.

Positioning:
Stand with your feet about six inches apart, holding a three-pound dumbbell in your right or left hand. Hold the dumbbell with your palm facing away from you, and form a slightly rounded L with your arm.

Exercise:
Bending at the waist and flexing your serratus and oblique muscles as hard as possible, lower your elbow and at the same time squeeze your side abdominal muscles as hard as possible. Place your other hand on your working oblique muscles so that you can feel the intensity of your peak contraction. While maintaining continual tension, return to the start position and repeat the movement until you have completed your set. Repeat the set for the other side of your body.

Tips:
Remember to flex your serratus and oblique muscles as you work. Be sure that it is your serratus and oblique muscles and not your arm that is doing the work. Throw your mind into that area and tell it to do the work. For an even more intense workout, twist your body to the

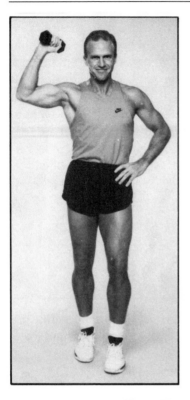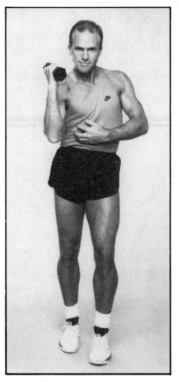

side until your elbow is nearly in line with your belly button.

Gym Alternative: You may perform this exercise on any gym pulley machine, including the lat–pull-down machine pulley. You may use a looped rope or a narrow bar. Set the weight at twenty pounds. If you are using the rope, intertwine your fingers around the rope, and work as described above. If you are using the narrow bar, intertwine your fingers around the center of the bar and work as described above.

Use of Weights:	Do not use any more than three-pound dumbbells or twenty pounds of weight in the gym. Any more weight will force your arms to do the work. You will defeat your purpose. (Don't be confused. Note that three-pound dumbbells are equivalent to twenty-pound weights because of the mechanical particulars of the machine versus the positioning of the dumbbell.)

THE OBLIQUE CRUNCH
Abdominal Exercise #7

This exercise develops, strengthens, and defines the oblique muscles. It also helps to develop the upper and lower abdominal areas.

Positioning:	Lie flat on your back on the floor and bend your knees. Place your feet together. Let your legs fall to one side, until your knees are as close to the floor as possible. Place your hands behind your head.
Exercise:	With your chest still facing straight to the ceiling, raise your shoulders off the floor as high as possible. Be sure to move up in a straight line and to lift from the chest, not from the neck. Repeat the movement until you have completed your set. Repeat the set for the other side of your body.

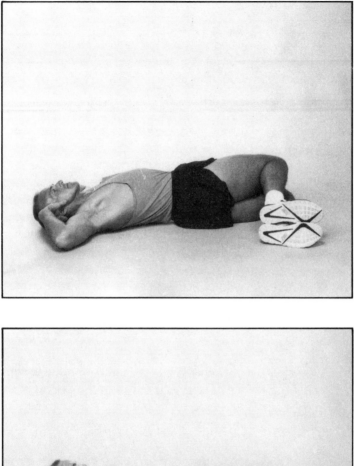

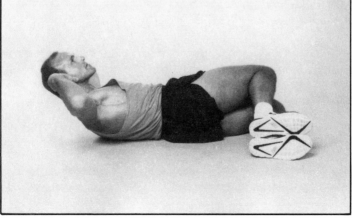

| Tips: | Beware of the temptation to pull on your neck. Keep your mind riveted on your oblique muscles as you work. |

| Gym Alternative: | You may perform this exercise by positioning yourself face upward on the hyperextension bench. Place your feet under the padded bar and lean back until your body is nearly parallel to the floor. Raise your body to one side until your elbow nearly touches the opposite knee. Now do the same movement for the other side of your body. Continue this alternate left-right-left-right movement until you have completed your set. |

| Use of Weights: | Do not use weights for the oblique crunch. You may use a ten- to twenty-five-pound plate if you are working on the hyperextension bench. However, do not use a weight until you can perform three sets of twenty-five repetitions without a weight. Then start with a five- or ten-pound plate, and gradually work your way up to twenty-five pounds. |

WHAT IF YOU CAN'T DO ONE EXERCISE, AND CAN'T DO THE ALTERNATIVE EITHER?

If you have back problems, and your doctor advises you not to perform one of the exercises, simply replace the forbidden exercise with any other abdominal exercise you can do, even if this means you will be doing three or four groups of, say, plain old crunches to make up for exercises you cannot do.

Where possible, it's a good idea to replace equivalent exercises—for example, those that stress upper abdominals for others that stress upper abdominals. The crunch can replace the sit-up, the reverse crunch can replace the leg-raise, and so on.

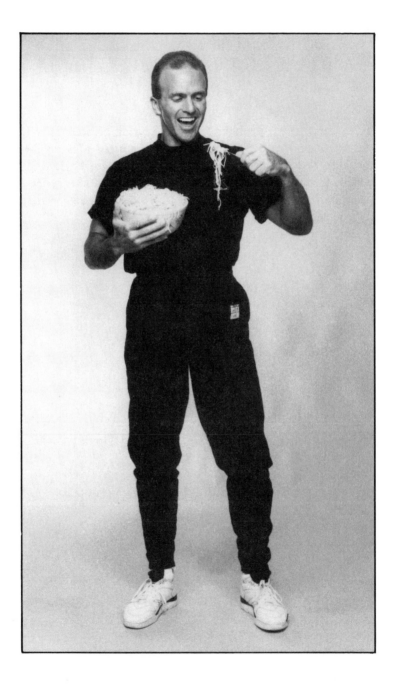

5

THE FAT-ATTACK
FOOD PLAN

In order to see progress, you will have to cooperate with the workout by eating properly. No diet is involved. This is simply a new way of thinking about food—for life. The bonus is, not only will you have a well-defined, muscular stomach, but improved health. Your cholesterol level will go down, as well as your blood pressure, and your energy level will go up, and all of this will happen without the sacrifice of delicious food. The only thing you'll be giving up is the unhealthy fat in your diet. But before you learn new fat-free eating habits, here are a few necessary basics about nutrition.

CALORIES

A calorie is the amount of energy required to raise the temperature of a gram of water one degree Celsius. How does this apply to food consumption? All food contains calories, or potential fuel for your body. Whenever you eat, you supply your body with fuel, or energy, so that you can move from point A to point B. The same way a car will not operate without fuel, your body would not function if you did not eat. In fact, if you did not supply your body with needed fuel (food), you would eventually starve to death. However, although an intake of calories is necessary for life, some calories are a poor food bargain, while others are a "deal." Here's why:

Fat Calories Versus Other Calories

There are three basic food groups: fats, proteins, and carbohydrates. Of the three, fat calories are the "fattest," the least desirable. Fat contains more calories per gram than do the other two food groups. Specifically, there are 4 calories per gram of carbohydrate and protein, but 9 calories per gram of fat.

But that's not the end of the "fatness" of fat calories. In one sense, fat calories really do go straight to your waist. You see, it takes little or no energy to digest fat calories; only about 3 percent of the energy of fat calories is used up in the digestion process. By comparison, it takes a lot of energy to digest protein and carbohydrate calories; about 15 percent of these calories are used up in the digestion process. Simply put, when you consume fat calories, they are quickly available for immediate use or storage as fat, and since most of us don't use them up, they go straight to favorite fat storage places on our bodies.

PROTEIN—
IT'S WHAT MUSCLES ARE MADE OF

Most body material is composed of protein: muscle, internal organs, blood, hair, and nails. Protein also plays an important role in regulating water balance in the body.

Protein is composed of twenty-two amino acids. Eight of these are produced naturally by the human body, but the other fourteen are not, and must be obtained from foods that contain them. These fourteen have come to be known as "essential amino acids." The foods that contain them include red meat, poultry, fish, milk, and milk products, and egg whites.

However, red meat and full-fat milk and milk products are high in fat as well as protein, so you should obtain your protein requirement from lower-fat proteins, such as white-meat poultry, fish, and egg whites. Fortunately, there is enough low-fat protein to enjoy life without feeling as if you're being deprived.

The body absorbs protein in small amounts—about twenty to thirty grams per meal. For this reason, it is inadvisable to consume more than that in one sitting. Excess protein is stored by the body in the form of fat, just as are any other excess calories. The ideal way to consume protein, then, is in three or more smaller portions a day, as opposed to one large portion a day.

CARBOHYDRATES—
THE FUEL FOR YOUR BODY

Carbohydrates provide energy not only for your body, but for your mind. If you've ever gone on one of those high-protein, low-carbohydrate diets, the first thing you probably noticed was that you became weak and irritable. Your body and mind are being deprived of life-sustaining energy.

When carbohydrates are ingested, they are immediately processed by the digestive system into glucose, or blood sugar. This glucose supplies the central nervous system with basic energy, together with all muscle tissue.

There are two types of carbohydrates: simple and complex. Simple carbohydrates have an undeserved bad reputation. They are said to give a quick energy boost and then a let-down. But this is only true if you consume them to the exclusion or the limitation of complex carbohydrates.

There is a time and place for simple carbohydrates. In fact, a good dose of certain simple carbohydrates (fruits) can give you a much needed energy boost. Even processed simple carbohydrates (jam, jelly, hard candy, etc.) have their proper place at times. They can help you resist indulging in high-fat foods, because in eating them you may satisfy a craving. By eating these seemingly forbidden foods, you may curb your appetite for high-fat foods, such as ice-cream, doughnuts, or chocolate. (Carbohydrates, even simple ones, have only 4 calories per gram. As you will recall, fats contain 9 calories per gram.)

It may surprise you to read that it is okay to consume simple processed carbohydrates in moderation. Consider also what is now common knowledge among health and nutrition experts: The body processes the sugar found in fruit in the same way it processes the sugar found in candy, jams, or jellies. The sugar in fruit (fructose, sucrose, and glucose) and the sugar in most candies and jams are virtually identical. They are both simple sugar molecules and are quickly digested. In both cases, the sugar is converted into glucose and used as an immediate source of energy. Either way, if you eat these on an empty stomach, you get a quick burst of energy and then a quick letdown.

Of course, it is always better to consume fruit, because fruit contains needed fiber and vitamins, whereas the sugar found in jams, jellies, and candy is commonly regarded as "empty calories." But are they really so empty?

Men and women report that because our fat-attack food plan allows them to have processed, low-fat sugar products, they are able to maintain their low-fat eating habits without feeling deprived. Allowing the consumption of these former food outlaws saves them from abandoning the low-fat eating plan. So if you have the urge for an occasional low-fat sweet, unless your doctor has instructed you otherwise, go for it.

Complex carbohydrates in the form of grains and vegetables are superior to simple carbohydrates. The molecular structure of these carbohydrates entails a gradual breakdown into glucose, which results in slowly released energy over a long period of time (up to four hours). You should make complex carbohydrates your dietary mainstay, and use unprocessed simple carbohydrates (fruits) as your backup, with processed simple carbohydrates as your binge-avoiding treat.

There is yet another food that can save you from indulging in high-fat bingeing: pretzels—both soft and hard. Pretzels are generally composed of processed complex carbohydrates (bleached flour) and are high in sodium—not the best nutritional deal on the market. However, they are not the worst deal either, because they contain many needed food nutrients, and supply energy for hours after consumption. If you have a strong desire for a "goody" and you decide to eat pretzels, you will be consuming virtually no fat (read the package to be sure). If sodium is a problem for you, you can always get low-sodium pretzels.

SODIUM—
NOT AS BAD AS MOST PEOPLE THINK

Sodium, in combination with potassium, helps to regulate body fluids and maintain the acid-alkali balance of the blood. The sodium-potassium combination is also responsible for helping our muscles to contract. Bodybuilders often deliberately allow their bodies to be depleted of sodium before a contest so that they can appear "ripped"; boxers or wrestlers often do the same in an effort to "make weight." In either case these athletes often find themselves in the predicament of having muscle cramps at the wrong time. Such episodes can cost them the contest. Insufficient sodium can also cause muscle shrinkage and intestinal gas.

Healthy people should not seek to totally eliminate sodium from their diet. In any case, this would be very difficult, since virtually everything we eat or drink contains some sodium. Tap water contains 10 milligrams of sodium per eight ounces, and club soda twenty-five milligrams for the same amount. Even an innocent slice of whole wheat bread contains 120 milligrams, while the desirable chicken breast contains 150 milligrams.

Since sodium holds up to fifty times its own weight in water, excessive sodium consumption can result in water retention. In fact, it is not unusual for people to carry from five to ten pounds of excess water in their bodies if they habitually consume extremely high sodium foods.

A healthy daily sodium intake range is between 1,500 and 2,500 milligrams. Foods that contain excessive sodium include canned, smoked, or pickled foods; many frozen dinners, including "diet" dinners; Chinese foods; pizza; frankfurters; and condiments such as table salt, ketchup, mustard, A-1 sauce, and Worcestershire sauce. These items contain a thousand or more milligrams of sodium per modest serving—and most people who use these condiments do not use them in moderation.

If you enjoy high-sodium foods, and if you have no problem with high blood pressure, plus you don't mind temporary water-weight gain obscuring your developing abdominals, from time-to-time, you may want to enjoy high-sodium foods. When you are finished, if you cut your sodium level to the advised amount for three to five days, you will eliminate any excess water, and find no harm has been done. In fact, it may be a good idea to forget all about monitoring your sodium while you are busy paying attention to fat grams. If you have to watch everything at once, you may become demoralized and want to abandon your program completely. It may be better to lose your fat first, and then drop your sodium intake in the last week of your program.

Water weight is not real weight. It's very temporary, and can be flushed out of your system in a matter of days. Fat weight, on the other hand, is very real. It sticks to your muscles and takes weeks to eliminate.

Water Flushes Out Excess Sodium

Ironically, water itself is a friend to water loss. The more water you drink, the less water you will retain. You will also retain less water while eating high-sodium foods if you drink a lot of water while eating. Drink a minimum of six 8-ounce glasses of plain (tap or bottled) water a day. It's a great way to keep your skin looking younger, and also gives your body a daily internal shower.

THE FAT-ATTACK FOOD PLAN

Now that you know the basic facts about food, it's time to plan your new style of eating. The quintessence of the plan is simple: Never consume more than 30 to 40 grams of fat in the course of a day. If you keep to this limit (and it won't be easy until you know where all the fat is hidden), you can be sure your excess body fat will melt away and your developing abdominals will be revealed.

Where's the Fat?

For your reference, here is a quick fat-detection list. However, you should get yourself a copy of *The Fat Gram Counter* (see bibliography) and/or a copy of *The Nutrition Almanac.* These books will be well worth the small investment.

One cup of each of the following fat bandits contains:

potato chips	60 grams of fat
roasted cashew nuts	64 grams of fat
rich ice-cream	23 grams of fat
regular ice-cream	14 grams of fat
whole milk	8 grams of fat

One ounce of the following fat bandits contains:

cream cheese	11 grams of fat
American cheese	9 grams of fat
cheddar cheese	9 grams of fat
Swiss cheese	8 grams of fat
part-skim mozzarella	5 grams of fat

Six ounces of the following fat bandits contain:

sausage	62 grams of fat
cooked spareribs	51 grams of fat
veal chop or cutlet	46 grams of fat
flank steak	32 grams of fat
round steak	26 grams of fat
ground regular beef	23 grams of fat
ground lean beef	20 grams of fat
very lean pork chop	20 grams of fat
cooked loin of lamb	16 grams of fat

The following items contain:

1 doughnut	27 grams of fat
1 tablespoon butter or margarine	12 grams of fat
1 tablespoon vegetable oil	14 grams of fat
1 tablespoon peanut butter	8 grams of fat
1 chocolate chip cookie	3 grams of fat

A slice of regular pizza contains about 6 grams of fat—not so bad if you love pizza. If you blot the top with a paper napkin, you take off at least 2 grams of the fat. It's okay to indulge in a slice or two once in a while.

What *Can* You Eat?

The answer is simple. Just about everything else, and that's a lot. You can eat white-meat chicken and turkey with the skin removed, and low-fat fish, such as flounder, tuna canned in water, sole, haddock, halibut, perch, pike, pollock, and snapper. You can have plenty of fresh or frozen fruits and vegetables, and best of all, you can have plenty of grains such as rice, pasta, and bran. Let's get into the details.

Eat Smaller Portions, But Eat More Often

If your goal is to lose weight, the worst thing you can do is eat nothing all day, and then consume one big meal at the end of the day. The body is a survival system. If more than four hours go by without food, your metabolism slows down in an effort to preserve energy and to help the body to survive. This means that while ordinarily you might burn 80 calories an hour talking on the telephone, you will now burn only 60 calories an hour. You could and should have eaten something earlier; you would have lost more weight.

Your goal is to feed your body scientifically so that you are not tired, you burn the maximum fat, and you are never hungry. The best way to do this is to eat more often than the traditional three times a day. The idea is to *eat often, but eat smaller portions than usual!* Every time you eat a little something, your metabolism speeds up in order to process the food taken in and release energy to you more promptly for use. Here is a sample eating plan. You don't have to think of these five eating sessions as meals. You can think of three as meals and two as snacks if you wish.

Meal #1 (Breakfast)

1 cup cold or hot cereal (bran, wheat, oat, or high-fiber)
   or 1 whole egg plus 2 or 3 egg whites
   or 1 bran muffin and 1 tablespoon jelly
   or 1 bagel and 1 tablespoon jelly

and

1 fruit or 6 ounces fruit juice (fruit is better than juice;
   it contains fiber, and leaves you feeling less hungry)

and

no-calorie beverage
   or skim milk if desired

Meal #2 (Snack)

2 fruits
   or 6 ounces low-fat cottage cheese or yogurt
   or 2 slices whole wheat toast and 1 tablespoon jelly

Meal #3 (Lunch)

6 to 8 ounces white-meat poultry or low-fat fish
2 cups vegetables
1 baked potato
   or 1 cup pasta with tomato sauce
   or 1 cup rice
large tossed salad with vinegar and spices

Meal #4 (Dinner)

6 to 8 ounces any low-fat protein (e.g. fish or chicken)
1 baked potato
    or 1 cup rice
    or 1 sweet potato
    or 1 yam
    or 1 cup pasta with tomato sauce
    or 2 ears corn on the cob
2 cups vegetables
1 large tossed salad
no-calorie beverage

Meal #5 (Late snack)

2 slices whole wheat toast with jelly
    or 1 bran muffin with jelly
    or 6 ounces low-fat cottage cheese on lettuce
    or 4 ounces tuna on lettuce with tossed salad

In addition to your five meals, you may consume any of the following vegetables in unlimited quantities whenever you are hungry:

asparagus	lettuce
bamboo shoots	mushrooms
green or yellow beans	mustard greens
brussels sprouts	okra
cauliflower	onions
celery	peppers—red or green
chard	spinach
collard	tomatoes
cucumber	turnips
endive	watercress
kale	

Limit your servings of corn, potatoes, yams, sweet potatoes, beets, beans to two servings a day. You should have
two to four fruits a day.

Never go hungry. Remember: Eat often and eat low-fat.
Do not allow yourself to feel deprived.

ONE KEY TO MAINTAINING YOUR LOW-FAT BODY—A *FREE WEEKLY EATING DAY!*

There's good news. Once you attain your weight goal, you
may eat anything you want one day per week, and in any
quantity. That's right. If you feel like it, you can eat half a
pizza, a big juicy red steak, and three scoops of ice cream.
As long as you do that only once a week, you will not gain
back the weight.

Once your body has been reoriented to a low-fat regi-
men, you make yourself sick if you overeat; your own body
will rebuke you into more moderate behavior. Even so,
when we say you may eat anything you want once a week,
once you reach your weight goal, we mean it. In fact, we
want you to do that. If you don't, you will eventually rebel
against restrictions and begin pigging out on a regular
basis.

WHAT IF YOU "LOSE IT" AND PIG OUT FOR DAYS AT A TIME?

If you "pig out" for more than one day, such as on
vacations or holidays, you'll have to give up one week of

free eating for each extra day you pigged out. For example, if you went on a vacation and ate like a pig for seven days, you would have to wait six weeks before taking the next free eating day. (Remember, one of the days was yours for the taking. You "stole" the other six and must pay for them now.) If you only pigged out for three days, you only have to wait two weeks to take advantage of your free eating day.

We don't recommend pigging out for an entire week. All hotels and resorts offer low-fat foods. You just have to know what to ask for. Where in the world can you not get a simple baked potato, or broiled fish with nothing on it, or plain white rice, or fresh fruit? Get a copy of *The Twelve-Minute Total-Body Workout,* which has an entire chapter on what to order from hotel menus, if you feel that you need help. (See the bibliography.)

WHAT ABOUT ALCOHOL?

If you drink, you must do it very moderately while trying to lose fat. Stick to light beer, white wine, champagne, or vodka with club soda or fruit juice. Drink no more than three drinks a week. You can spread them out over the week, or have them all in one day. After you reach your goal, you can over-indulge on your free eating day if you wish.

REVIEW: RULES OF THE EATING GAME

- Consume low-fat protein three times a day.
- Never consume more than 30 to 40 grams of fat in one day.
- Have two to four fruits a day.
- Eat five times a day
- In addition, eat whenever you are hungry, but only unlimited complex carbohydrates.
- Don't punish yourself with over-diligence to sodium unless your doctor has mandated that you do so. Water retention is temporary. Pretzels are a high-sodium low-fat treat.
- If you are so inclined, indulge in "sweets" such as jams, jellies and low-fat candies once in a while. This may help you not to feel deprived, and may encourage you to keep your intake of fat low.
- Be sure to eat at least three cups of vegetables daily.
- Once you reach your weight goal, eat anything you want one day a week.
- Get a fat gram counter and become aware of fat in general.

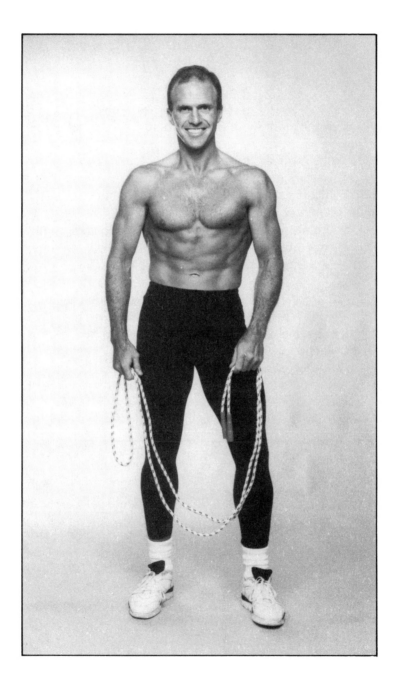

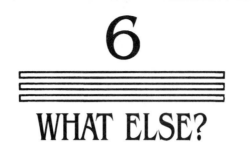

6

WHAT ELSE?

You now know how to exercise your abdominals. You understand the basic principles of low-fat eating. Is there anything else you should do if you want a near-perfect stomach and basic good health? Yes.

Your abdominal routine will result in the formation of a strong, muscular, well-defined stomach area. Your low-fat eating plan will ensure the reduction of fat all over your body—especially where fat tends to accumulate most on men, the abdominal area. But in order to help your body to burn fat continually, some aerobics are a must. Aerobic activities raise your metabolism for hours after you perform them, and help ensure yourself a healthy heart and strong lungs.

We're not talking about marathon running or triathalon competition. We're talking about three to six twenty- to thirty-minute sessions of something as calming and enjoyable as riding a stationary bicycle. In fact, it was recently discovered that aerobic sessions of even ten to fifteen minutes are effective in burning fat. What's more, we're not going to ask you to go at a mad pace. In order to burn the maximum amount of fat, all you have to do is get your pulse rate up to between 60 and 80 percent of its maximum, and maintain that level for the duration of your workout. In this range, your body converts stored body fat into fuel. You literally "burn it off." Your tongue does not have to be hanging out, and you do not have to be gasping for breath. In fact, if these signs are apparent, you can be sure that you're working too hard.

FIGURING OUT YOUR IDEAL AEROBIC PULSE RANGE

How can you tell when you're in the ideal fat-burning pulse range? First, you have to figure out your maximum aerobic pulse rate. You do this by subtracting your age from 220. This is your maximum pulse rate—the rate that would leave you with your tongue hanging out, gasping for breath. Now to find your ideal range, multiply the maximum rate by 0.60. This will give you the floor rate of 60 percent of your maximum rate. Use the same system to find your 70 percent and 80 percent rates.

You can find your pulse by simply placing your index and middle fingers on your wrist or neck. Time yourself on a watch with a second hand, for six seconds. Count the beat of your pulse within that time frame. After six seconds, stop and get a number. Then add a zero to whatever that number is. For example, if the number is thirteen, add a zero to determine that your pulse rate is 130.

What if you don't feel like figuring out your pulse rate every time you engage in an aerobic activity? Many people never check their pulse rate. They learn to "know" their bodies. If you are one of these people, your rule of thumb is simple. After about five to ten minutes, you should break into a sweat. As mentioned above, you should not be gasping for breath. This is your fat-burning range. Joyce never checks her pulse rate. And as you can see, she's successful at keeping fat off her body.

SELECTING AN AEROBIC ACTIVITY

There is such a variety of aerobic activities to choose from, that there's no reason for anyone to be miserable. Do what you like. If you hate riding the stationary bicycle, then run at an easy pace. If you hate running, use the stair machine. If you can't stand the stair machine, then walk fast. If you don't like walking, then use the Nordic Track machine. If that doesn't excite you, jump rope. If none of those things appeal to you, swim. In short, do what you enjoy.

What? You don't enjoy any of these things? Then choose the least of all evils; do something that is convenient for you.

For example, if you live in a city and take public transportation to work, why not walk instead of ride. If you can walk to work in between twenty and forty minutes, put on your running shoes and go.

If you like to watch a certain television program in the evening, ride the stationary bicycle while you're watching. The time will go by painlessly, and you will have accomplished your aerobic workout for the day.

If you go to a gym that has a stair machine or a treadmill, before you leave, jump on one or the other for twenty to thirty minutes. There will be people around you to distract your attention and, before you know it, you've finished the exercise.

BREAKING IN GENTLY TO
AEROBIC ACTIVITIES

If you are an "old hand" at aerobic activities, you can ignore this section. If you are new at aerobics, it's a good idea to break in gently—otherwise you may become discouraged and want to quit altogether.

Week 1:	three to five minutes
Week 2:	five to seven minutes
Week 3:	seven to ten minutes
Week 4:	ten to fifteen minutes
Week 5:	fifteen to twenty minutes
Week 6:	twenty to twenty-five minutes
Week 7:	twenty-five to thirty minutes

The idea is to begin at the lower end of the scale and work your way to the higher end each week. For example, on your first workout day of Week 1, perform your aerobic activity for three minutes. On your first workout day of Week 2, you exercise for four minutes. On your third, fourth, and fifth weeks (depending upon how many days you do aerobics), you perform for longer.

KEEPING IT UP "ON THE ROAD"

Few of us have hum-drum routines that are never interrupted by travel. Many of us are required to leave our home for days or even weeks at a time in order to conduct necessary business. So the question arises: Is it possible to maintain your abdominal workout, stick to your low-fat eating plan, and perform your aerobic activities while traveling?

Yes. Yes. Yes. That's the beauty of this workout. As you've already noticed, you need little or no equipment for the abdominal workout. What about the weights? No problem. Even if you've advanced to using weights with your workout, while you're traveling, if you simply exert more pressure (continual tension) on your abdominal muscles as you work out, you will more than make up for the lack of weights. Then when you get back home, you can resume the use of weights.

For those of you who are compulsive, however (we say this with tongue in cheek), and feel that you want to use weights even as you travel, you may order fill-up water weights (they go up to six pounds) by calling CAEF Inc. at 1-800-635-8132.

What about aerobics on the road? That's as simple as carrying a child's jump rope with you. You can jump rope in the morning, the moment you get up, while you watch the morning news on television. Don't worry about shaking the ceiling below you. People have jumped rope in hotel or motel rooms all across America with no problem. Fortunately, hotels are built in such a way that the impact of rope jumping is well absorbed by the construction of the floor and ceiling.

If you don't like rope jumping, you can do jumping jacks in your room, or you can take a brisk walk or run outdoors. If your hotel has a gym, you can take advantage of the equipment they have—stationary bicycle, stair machine, treadmill, or what have you.

As far as diet is concerned, there's no excuse to throw all caution to the wind just because you're dining out. Hotel menus including room service as a rule have excellent low-fat choices. If you review the principles of low-fat eating as described in Chapter 5, you'll know just what to order and what to avoid, or you can pick up a copy of *The*

Twelve-Minute Total-Body Workout, which has a more detailed chapter on selecting from hotel menus, including room service, for low-fat eating "on the road." (See the bibliography.)

MAINTAINING YOUR ABDOMINALS FOREVER

How can you ensure that you will never again have a "gut" that ruins your overall appearance? Adhere to the basic exercise program described in this book. Do you ever get a vacation from working out? Yes. You may take off one week every six months without fear of the consequences. Your body will jump right back into shape after a week of returning to the workout.

If you work out diligently but slowly let your low-fat eating plan slip, you may find yourself gaining a few pounds, and see those pounds translated into fat lying right on top of your gorgeous stomach muscles. Don't despair. The muscles are still there, just temporarily obscured under the fat. You can't see them as well as before, but all you have to do is pound hard on your stomach, and you'll be quickly reassured. When you want to see the muscles more clearly and show them off to the world, all you have to do is lose the excess fat by returning to the simple gut-busting program spelled out for you here.

No matter what you do, men, don't drop the workout. If you do, you'll have to work to regain muscularity again. If you do work out, but decide to pig out every day and get as fat as you please, at least your muscles will be there waiting for you when you come to your senses, if you've stayed with the exercise program.

While we're on the subject, there's good news for those who do lay off working out completely. It will take you only about <u>one-third the time</u> it originally took you to get in shape? Why is this so? Muscles seem to remember. Once they have been developed, even if thereafter they are neglected, they are ready to make a comeback. In a sense, you have "muscles in the bank." If it took you three months to develop your abdominals, and you maintained them for a year and then quit for a year, and then start working out again, this time it will take only a month to get them back. (Remember, of course, that you will not see them until the excess fat has also been removed from that area.)

WHAT'S MISSING?

You've developed your abdominal muscles. Everyone can see them because you've followed the low-fat eating plan and you've even done some aerobics. You feel great. Guess what. We're not satisfied. We know how much better you will look and feel if you dare to exercise the other seven body parts that are crying for attention. Your chest, shoulders, back, arms (biceps and triceps), and legs (thighs and calves) are feeling neglected. They cry for a workout that will put them on a par with your stomach. And that workout is not difficult at all.

If you want to go the extra mile, get a copy of *The Fat-Burning Workout*. Don't be put off by the woman on the cover (Joyce Vedral). The workout is one used by champion male and female bodybuilders before contests, to achieve total body hardness without bulk and with the elimination of all fat. The workout in that book takes twenty, thirty, or forty minutes, depending on your ambition, and it covers all body parts. Kent has been using it for months, and even trained the New Jersey Devils hockey team with it—and they loved it! If you want bigger muscles, get a copy of *Now or Never*.

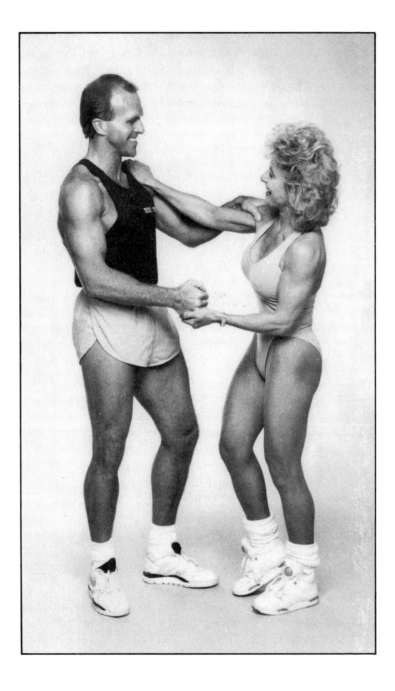

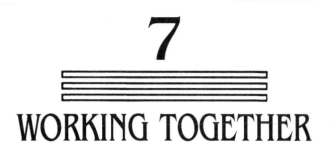

7

WORKING TOGETHER

This is a chapter about "partnering." If you wish, you may do your abdominal workout, and follow your low-fat eating plan with your spouse, girlfriend or companion. In the case of the abdominal workout, this is very easy, because the only difference in the workout is the amount of weight used in the exercises that require weight. There is also one very important upper abdominal exercise that cannot be done alone, so if you are lucky enough to have a partner, take advantage of it.

Some people enjoy working alone. In fact, some people consider the presence of another while working out a hindrance and a potential drain of energy. But if you are among those who enjoy and appreciate company when working out—because it makes the workout seem less arduous—then by all means pair up.

Since little or no equipment is needed for the abdominal

workout, and because little space is needed, you can work with your partner just about anywhere in your home. In fact, if you're accustomed to wedging your feet under a piece of heavy furniture while doing sit-ups, you are now even free of that strategem, because, as shown in the photograph (see p. 93) you can interlace your legs with your partner's.

FLOOR SIDEBEND
Partnering Exercise #1

This exercise develops, tightens, and tones the upper abdominal area, and also challenges the lower abdominal area.

Positioning:	Lie on the floor on your right side, with your body in as straight a line as possible. Keep your knees together and clasp your hands behind your head.
Exercise:	Have your partner straddle your legs, and place both of her hands on your hip-thigh area. Flexing your oblique muscles as hard as possible, lift your upper body sideways, as high as possible. Return to the start position and, without resting, repeat the movement until you have completed your set. Repeat the set for the other side of your body. Now quickly change positions so your partner can do the exercise. Continue to switch positions until you have both performed three sets.

Tips:

Remember to apply continual tension to your entire abdominal area, especially to your oblique muscles. Do not pull on your neck. Raise yourself with the power of your oblique muscles.

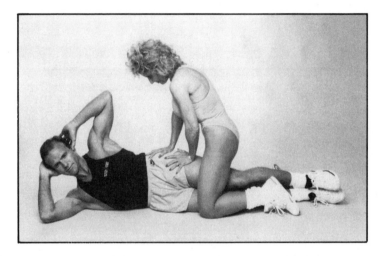

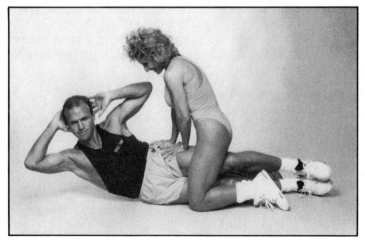

SIT-UP
Partnering Exercise #2

This exercise strengthens and defines the upper abdominal area. The lower abdominal area is also strengthened.

Positioning: Both partners lie flat on their backs with hands behind their head and with knees bent, legs interlaced.

Exercise: Using a fluid movement and flexing your entire abdominal area, especially the upper portion, simultaneously rise to the full sit-up position. You will enjoy the anchoring effect of the interlaced leg position. Without resting, and applying continual tension, return to the start position and repeat the movement until you have completed your set.

Tips: This is fun—so much fun that you may find yourself laughing and then merely twisting into the sit-up position. You can have a good time, but don't forget to flex your abdominal area and to maintain good form. Do not lurch off the floor or simply drop to the start position. Maintain a steady, fluid movement.

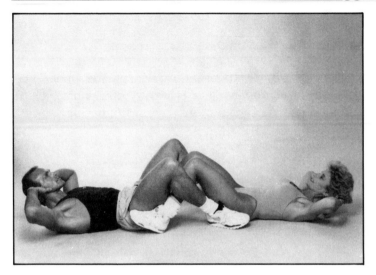

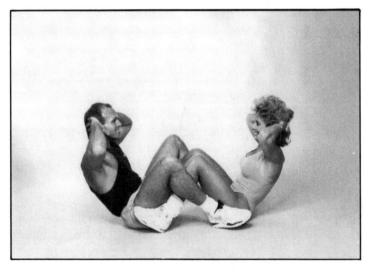

V-UP
Partnering Exercise #3

This exercise strengthens and develops the upper and lower abdominal areas. It is extremely challenging. Don't be discouraged if you cannot maintain balance in the beginning.

Positioning: Lie flat on your back with your heads in opposite directions. Your waists should be lined up, and you should be about a foot away from each other. Place your feet together, with your knees slightly bent, and extend your hands straight out behind you.

Exercise: Alternating from person to person, do the V-up. Simultaneously raise your upper and lower body by bringing your arms forward and raising your legs. Keep your feet together as you move. Raise both lower and upper body as high as you can go and, in complete control, return to the start position. Repeat the movement until you have completed your set.

Tips: This is a difficult exercise, and you may feel awkward at first as you both attempt to get into the V position. Laugh, but keep going. Remember your goal—a firm, well-defined abdominal area.

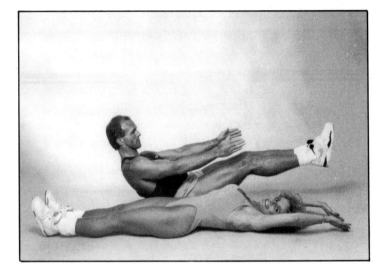

CRUNCH
Partnering Exercise #4

This exercise strengthens and develops the upper abdominal area.

Positioning: Lie flat on your backs on the floor, feet facing each other. Interlace your legs as in the partnering sit-up (see photograph on page 93).

Exercise: Simultaneously rise to the crunch position, performing the exercise as described on page 48.

Tips: If you are doing a true crunch, you will not be able to make full eye contact with your partner when you rise to the crunch position. Do not let this tempt you into raising more than your shoulders off the floor. If you find yourself unable to resist the urge to sit up farther, change positions and do the crunch side by side, heads in the same direction.

LEG RAISE
Partnering Exercise #5

This exercise strengthens and develops the lower abdominal area.

Positioning: Lie on the floor with your heads in opposite directions, side by side. You should be about a foot apart and your waists should be approximately lined up with each other.

Exercise: Alternately lower and raise your legs in a see-saw motion. The rhythm of this movement will create energy to perform the workout. Perform the exercise as described on pages 50–51.

Tips: If you find it distracting to alternately raise and lower your legs, you may raise and lower them in synchrony. If one of you works faster than the other, you will soon be out of sync. Do *not* slow down for your partner. However, the slow partner may speed up to catch up.

KNEE-IN
Partnering Exercise #6

This exercise develops, strengthens, and defines the lower abdominal area. It also challenges the upper abdominal area and the oblique muscles.

Positioning: Lie flat on your backs, side by side, with your heads in opposite directions. You should be about a foot apart and your waists should be lined up with each other.

Exercise: Alternately draw your knees as far into your chest as possible. As one person returns to the start position, the other is pulling the knees to the chest. Continue this alternating draw-extend movement until you have each completed your set. The alternate movement will spark energy for the workout, and provide some fun, too. The exercise will seem to go quickly. Follow the directions on page 53.

Tips: If you find it distracting to alternate the leg-in movement—because you are rising up to look at each other—perform it side by side, either alternately or simultaneously.

THE SERRATUS PULL
Partnering Exercise #7

This exercise strengthens and develops the serratus muscles and helps to define the oblique muscles.

Positioning: Stand side by side, facing a mirror and holding a dumbbell in your right arm, which is in an L position.

Exercise: Perform the exercise movements simultaneously, bending at the waist and crunching forward. Be sure to let your serratus and oblique muscles do the work. You may place your free hand on your working muscles. This "in sync" crunching movement looks pretty in the mirror. Follow the directions on page 58.

Tips: If you do not have a mirror, you may both serve as mirror for the other by performing the exercise face to face.

WHAT IF ONE PARTNER CANNOT KEEP UP?

Suppose your partner can only do fifteen repetitions per set, while you can do twenty-five. This is not a problem. She can take advantage of the time you are working, to enjoy a few seconds more of a rest. Since she is not as strong as you, she will need the time.

In some cases, it will be the man who cannot keep up with the woman. In abdominal exercises, it is quite common to see women out-perform men. The explanation for this is simple: Abdominal exercises require little or no weight and high repetitions. Women are notorious champions when it comes to stamina. However, if the two of you were training with weights, it would be another matter. The man would quickly surpass the woman because, in general, men build larger muscles than do women because of a naturally higher level of the male hormone testosterone.

In addition, stamina depends on previous conditioning, general health, genetics, and a host of other things. The idea is not to get bogged down in the competition, but to use it as an impetus to spur each other on.

If your partner is slower than you are, great! Take that time to do more repetitions and get a more intense workout.

LOW-FAT EATING PARTNERSHIP

It's great to have a nutrition partner. Changing your eating habits alone can be difficult, but with someone working with you, it becomes more like a challenging game.

If you are married or living together, nutrition partnership makes dieting so simple. No one feels punished and no one is put out by being the only one forced to eat certain foods.

If you do not live together but share frequent meals, nutrition partnership is equally important. You can cook for each other, following the guidelines in Chapter 6, or you can eat out together, again following the guidelines in Chapter 6. No one will feel deprived.

WHAT IS THE DIFFERENCE IN THE WOMAN'S DIET?

Not much, I'm happy to say. The only real difference is, instead of being allowed 30 to 40 grams of fat a day, women are allowed only 20 to 30. The rest is basically the same. This means that women can eat as much fresh or frozen free vegetables as they please. However, most women will naturally eat less than will men during the course of a day. Why is this so? First of all, the man is probably taller than the woman, and has more muscles to begin with. His added height and muscularity raise his metabolism and his maintenance caloric needs, and he will naturally eat a little more.

Fortunately, with this food plan, you don't have to count calories—just grams of fat. I do not advise eating three pounds of pasta per meal—keep to the general guidelines of the meal plan presented in Chapter 5. Then, once you reach your goal, you can "pig out" once a week.

A FINAL NOTE

It's not okay to be content with just an abdominal workout. Ideally, you should make the effort to get your entire body in shape so that your posture improves and you wind up looking ten years younger. If you and your partner want to go a step farther, pick up a copy of *The Fat-Burning Workout, Now or Never* or *The Twelve-Minute Total-Body Workout* (see bibliography).

Let me know how you're doing. Write to me at the following address. If you wish a response, be sure to include a stamped, self-addressed envelope:

> Joyce L. Vedral
> P.O. Box 7433
> Wantagh, NY 11793-0433

The bench pictured on page 47 is an exercise bench that can be used to do flat, incline and decline exercises, and, as seen, incline sit-ups. If you wish to purchase this bench, send a check for $149.98 to Joyce Vedral at the above P.O. Box. You will pay United Parcel Service shipping charges C.O.D. Unfortunately, we cannot ship to Canada at this time. If you wish to pay the U.P.S. charges ahead of time, for easier delivery, add $20, for a total price of $169.98.

Bibliography

Katahn, Martin, Ph.D., and Jamie Pope-Cordle, M.S., R.D. *The T-Factor Fat Gram Counter.* New York: W.W. Norton & Company, 1989.

Kirshbaum, John (ed). *The Nutrition Almanac.* New York: McGraw-Hill, 1989.

Natow, Annette B., Ph.D., R.D., and Jo-Ann Heslin, M.A., R.D., *The Fat Attack Plan.* New York: Pocket Books, 1990.

Reynolds, Bill, and Joyce Vedral, Ph.D. *Supercut: Nutrition for the Ultimate Physique.* Chicago: Contemporary Books, 1987.

Vedral, Joyce, Ph.D., *Now or Never.* New York: Warner Books, 1986.

Vedral, Joyce, Ph.D. *The Twelve-Minute Total-Body Workout.* New York: Warner Books, 1989.

Vedral, Joyce, Ph.D. *The Fat-Burning Workout.* New York: Warner Books, 1991.

Vedral, Joyce, Ph.D. *Bottoms Up!* New York: Warner Books, 1993.

Vedral, Marthe Simone, and Joyce L. Vedral, Ph.D. *The College Dorm Workout.* New York: Warner Books, 1994.

VIDEOS BY JOYCE VEDRAL, Ph.D.

The Fat-Burning Workout, Volume I. (The regular workout.) New York: Time-Life Inc., 1992.

The Fat-Burning Workout, Volume II. (The intensity and insanity workouts.) New York: Time-Life Inc., 1992.

In most video stores or call 1-800-433-6769.

COMING SOON FOR MEN

Vedral, Joyce, Ph.D. *Top Shape.* New York: Warner Books, 1995.